JOANNA HALL'S
WALKACTIVE
PROGRAMME

THE SIMPLE YET REVOLUTIONARY WAY TO TRANSFORM YOUR BODY, FOR LIFE

JOANNA HALL
WITH LUCY ATKINS

piatkus

PIATKUS

First published in Great Britain in 2013 by Piatkus
Reprinted 2013, 2014
Copyright © Joanna Hall 2013
The moral right of the author has been asserted.
Walkactive is a registered trademark of Joanna Hall.

A CIP catalogue record for this book is available from the British Library.

ISBN 978-0-7499-5957-9

Designed and illustrated by D.R. ink. www.d-r-ink.com
Printed and bound in Great Britain by Butler Tanner and Dennis Ltd
Exercise photography © Dan Welldon

MIX
Paper from
responsible sources
FSC® C023561

Piatkus
An imprint of
Little, Brown Book Group
100 Victoria Embankment
London EC4Y 0DY

An Hachette UK Company
www.hachette.co.uk
www.piatkus.co.uk

Thank you to Casall for providing the T-shirts for the studio exercise shots and to Merrell for providing the shoes.

Picture credits
All photographs © Dan Welldon (p.20 courtesy of *Country Walking* magazine) except for p.70 ©Steve Debenport Imagery/iStock; p.95 © snapphoto/iStock; p.100 © digitalskillet/iStock; p.110 © Monkey Business Images/ Shutterstock

Important: Before starting any new activity discuss your plans with your doctor to ensure any conditions specific to you are accommodated.

ACKNOWLEDGEMENTS

Thinking back, I realise that I first began to create and develop Walkactive when I was pregnant with our daughter, Isabella. This was the catalyst. I wanted something that really worked for me – my posture, my body shape, my health, my confidence, my fitness, as well as my headspace at a time of tremendous change. So not only did I give birth to our beautiful, fun-loving daughter, but also to Walkactive! My first thank you therefore goes to Isabella – whose arrival not only started a whole new wonderful chapter and adventure in our lives but also prompted the development of Walkactive – thank you Poppet.

Throughout my career I have been blessed to have come in touch with so many lovely people from all walks of life. I've been humbled by some of the experiences we have shared, and I never cease to find the journey that starts to unfold as an individual progresses on their Walkactive journey deeply rewarding, motivating and inspiring. I cannot express how joyful and energising it is to continue to create and develop my Walkactive programmes. For this I want to say THANK YOU to all of our clients for starting on the Walkactive journey and for sharing your successes and stories, whatever your starting point – young, old, male, female, fit or those who've previously been inactive. I really look forward to sharing more with you. And especially to my own London Walkactive course participants, who have shared glorious moments of 'open ankles' and fabulous Ab Js – the weather may not always be brilliant sunshine but my journey with you has always been sunny and very rewarding, thank you.

To all my team at JHHQ, I couldn't do it without you. Lisa – thank you for our great working relationship and ... giving up your glass of Merlot on a Friday afternoon in the office as there is just too much to be done! To all in my Walkactive Trainer team: Trisha, Fiona, Sophie LW, Charlie, Keir, Rolande, Paula, Jo B, Debbie, Karen F, Angela T, Alice, Sarah D, Jen, Sarah P and Sybil, and especially my Elite Walkactive Trainers, Jo D and Ange F – thank you for your fabulous delivery of the 6Es! Thanks also to all the fabulous venues we work with, both in the UK and internationally; there are too many to mention here but we are grateful for the relationships and the support you have given us.

Lucy Atkins: thank you for letting me talk you into helping me write this book, I'm so glad you said yes. Thanks for keeping me on track, and for being so patient, diligent and committed in helping me communicate, inspire and educate through my work – you have been so great at this. It's been a joy – stressful timelines too – but a joy, thank you!

Thank you to Judith Murray, my literary agent, and all at Greene & Heaton, especially Claudia. Thanks too, to my publishers, Piatkus – especially Anne Lawrance, Jillian Stewart and Zoe Goodkin, and to my designer, Sian, at D.R.ink.: thank you for all your creativity. Thanks also to Noelle Shine at Palette Beauty, to Casall and Merrell for providing clothing and footwear for some of our photoshoots, and, of course, to the photographer Dan Welldon – your attention to detail and creative mind have so helped bring my words and training methods to life visually (but more about you later).

To David Greene and his team: a big thank you for the opportunity – I still need to work on that 'open ankle' though! To Darren James and his team at South Bank University's Sports Performance laboratory, thanks for your analysis and enthusiasm for my Walkactive technique. To Dr Tim Evans, thank you for your support for my work which started all those years ago with your amazing success with my programmes – time flies! To Charles and Allan, thank

you – you inspire, you listen, you share. To my dear girlfriends – to wine, laughter and friendships, thank you for being there.

And just as my first thank you was for my daughter Isabella, my last thank you is for my husband, Dan Welldon (I said I'd come back to you!) – for your incredible support, even when I'm tired and ratty! You have been encouraging me to write this book for SO long – so this is for you with all my thanks and all my love.

Your free Walkactive audio coaching session

To get you off to a flying start, Joanna Hall has recorded an exclusive 30-minute audio coaching session for readers. Once you have familiarised yourself with the basics of her Walkactive technique (see Chapter Two), you can simply download the session to your smartphone or portable MP3 player, put on your shoes, and head off for your first walk! For more information on how to access your free download, go to **www.joannahall.com**.

ABOUT THE AUTHOR

Joanna Hall, MSc (Sports Science), is a highly respected fitness professional. She has written twelve fitness books translated into six languages; is the producer and presenter of four fitness DVDs; has received over two million YouTube hits for her online exercise clips; was ITV's resident Diet and Fitness expert for three years, and has worked with the Royal Navy, the All Party Parliamentary Health Select Committee, multi-million-pound corporations, schools and celebrities.

Joanna Hall devised and founded Walkactive in 2008. She now presents and teaches her Walkactive Technique Programme and Intelligent Exercise System both in the UK and internationally through courses, residential programmes, one-day workshops, training camps and bespoke services. She is currently developing a series of educational support materials, including an audio coaching session for beginners (see opposite) and *Joanna Hall's Introduction to Walkactive Instructional DVD* to accompany her Walkactive programmes. See the website for details. **www.joannahall.com**

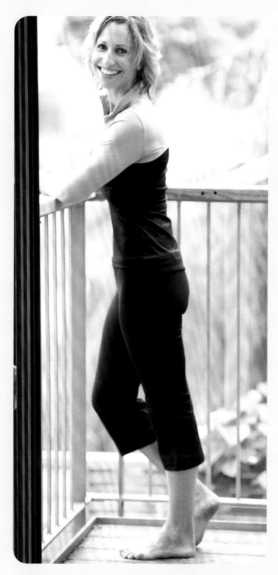

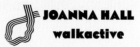

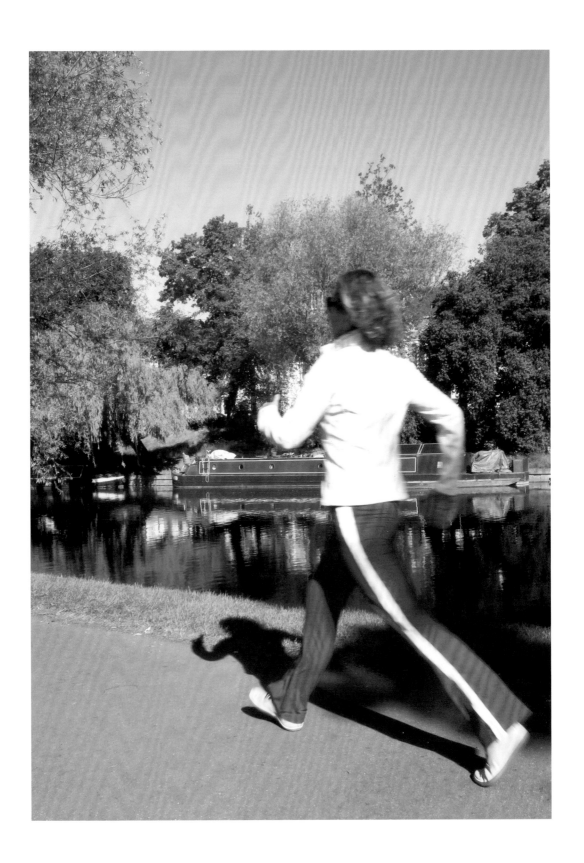

CONTENTS

INTRODUCTION

You think you know how to walk, don't you? Well, I have news for you – you almost certainly don't!

You may have been taught to play a great backhand in tennis or to perfect your golf swing, but I bet nobody has ever taught you how to walk correctly. Quite simply, the vast majority of us walk *wrong.* We use the wrong muscles, in the wrong way and at the wrong time – and we lose out on the amazing body benefits of walking, potentially causing ourselves all sorts of physical problems while we're at it.

Walking is the simplest of movements; it is the foundation of all our daily activity. And I'm going to teach you how to do it right, so that you can transform your body. Yes, I am serious. I'm going to teach you how to walk!

I call my method Walkactive because it is an active way to radically change your body, your health, your fitness, your mind – your entire life – for good. You may already spend a fair amount of time on your feet – commuting, shopping, chasing after children, or walking the dog. But wouldn't it be revolutionary if you used every single step to lose inches, tone up and slim down? With Walkactive, that's exactly what you'll do. You will also dramatically improve your posture, joints and health. And best of all, you'll *transfer* these amazing benefits to all aspects of your life – you'll gain confidence, *joie de vivre* and energy. This isn't temporary – it will last because you'll Walkactive for the rest of your life.

You may be thinking, 'Hang on a minute! I walk a lot already – and it makes no difference. The only thing that would change my body is boot camp or marathon running.' Well, it's understandable that you think that way. Right now, instead of using every muscle in your body really effectively as you walk, you are relying on a few 'old favourites' to do the hard work. You are therefore missing out on enormous calorie-burning, shaping and toning opportunities. You are also throwing your body out of alignment, leaving it unbalanced and strained. (If you aren't already experiencing problems such as back or joint pain, you may well do so eventually.) And that's why you're not seeing results from walking.

I'm going to teach you how to put one foot in front of the other so that – literally with every step – your body is toning up, elongating, growing fitter, slimmer, trimmer, more elegant and better aligned. I'm going to show you – in four simple stages – how to work your whole body, from the deep internal connective tissues outwards.

When you walk 'right' – and by the end of this book you will be doing that – you look and feel like a million dollars. Your muscles pull together and elongate, 'shrink-wrapping' themselves around your new, taut inner framework. You immediately look more fluid and energetic. Almost as soon as you start Walkactive, people will say to you, 'Have you lost weight?' or 'Wow, you look well!'

You'll quickly see other benefits too: your skin tone will improve, as will your general outlook. But that's not all. You will also be giving yourself a less visible gift – your health. Walkactive can lower your chance of future problems such as heart disease or high blood pressure; it can improve your cholesterol levels, your mobility and your ability to resist or recover from illness. It can also tackle, and even prevent, mood issues such as depression or anxiety. It may even help you to live longer. In short, Walkactive is good for your head, your heart *and* your bottom!

So, how do I know that Walkactive works? Quite simply, I've seen it happen – over and over again, with hundreds and hundreds of my clients. Absolutely anyone, regardless of their body shape, ability, age, life stage or fitness level can Walkactive. (My oldest client is ninety, though she says she feels twenty years younger since she started Walkactive.) I've worked with celebrities, elite athletes, the

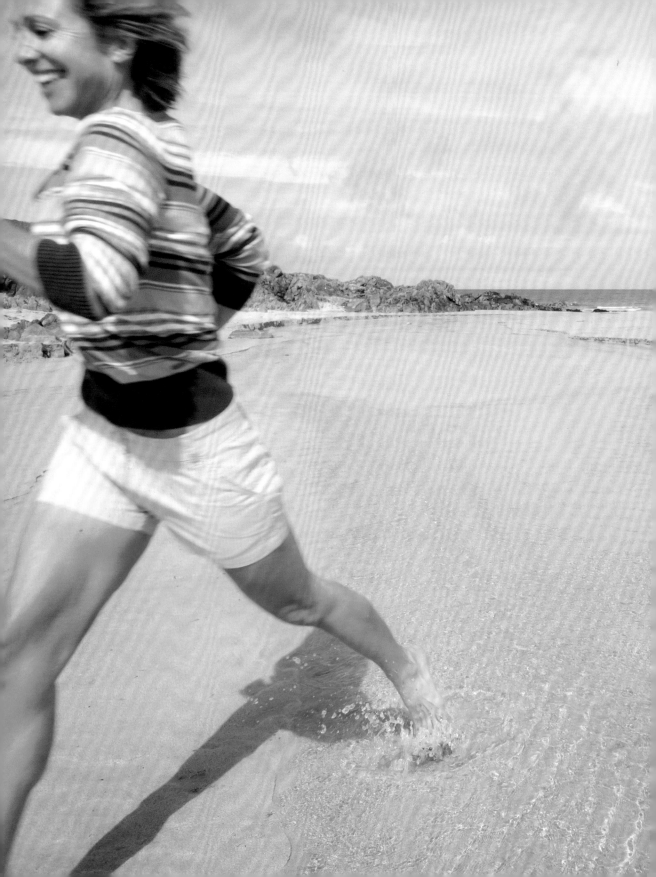

military, school-children, whole families and people recovering from illness or injury. I've seen people lose up to five inches around the waist in just four weeks. I've seen those who have struggled with their weight for years shrink to their ideal size in just a few months – and stay there, for the long term. I've seen 'non exercisers' blossom into dedicated, delighted walkers. I've seen top athletes boost their performance and recover from injuries, and fitness fanatics achieve new heights. In short, I've seen Walkactive change lives, over and over again. That's why you'll find lots of case studies and comments in this book – we have changed the names but these are *real* people talking about what Walkactive has done for them.

This isn't another stressful regime that you'll pick up, try for a bit, then drop. I'm not going to ask you to set foot in a gym, or set aside an hour three times a week to drag yourself out for 'exercise'. I'm simply going to teach you how to walk right in your daily life – and transform yourself by doing so. It really is as simple as that. So, are you raring to go? I hope so – because it's time to Walkactive!

'As a mother of four I've always been a regular exerciser. I've tried anything and everything, from military fitness, to yoga to gym sessions four times a week. But I've never seen results like this before. My stomach is flatter, my waist trimmer, my bottom has lifted, my legs have slimmed down and my clothes fit me like never before. My husband says I haven't looked this good since our wedding. I'm always telling people to try Walkactive. It's doable, it's fun – and it really works.'

JESSICA, 48, WALKACTIVE CLUB MEMBER

CHAPTER ONE

WALK RIGHT – WALKACTIVE

'This has been an amazing thing for my body – I really can feel the intelligent exercise working on me from the inside out!'

Before I teach you exactly how to walk right, I want you to learn a little bit about the science behind my technique – to understand exactly what it is you are doing *wrong* as you walk, and why Walkactive is walking 'right'. This is your first vital Walkactive step. It will help you to appreciate why Walkactive is different and why it will connect you with your body, bringing radical results. So don't be tempted to skip this chapter – this knowledge and science is crucial.

You may be wondering if Walkactive is right for you? To find out, ask yourself whether any of the following applies to you:

- You walk a reasonable amount every day, but while you feel healthier your body never changes.
- You experience back discomfort or pain after completing a walk.
- When walking fast or doing a longer-distance walk you notice discomfort in your back.
- Your knees sometimes feel sore from walking.

'I'm not a natural exerciser, but I knew I had to start doing something so I went to a one-day workshop with Joanna. It was hard to master the technique at first, but even after just seventy-five minutes I had glimmers of a gliding sensation with every step I took. I'm not saying it was perfect, but my body and the way it was moving felt amazing – and in such a short time.'

CHRIS, 28, ATTENDED A ONE-DAY INTRODUCTORY WORKSHOP

- You like the idea of getting fit, healthy and losing weight with walking, but are sceptical as to whether it could ever bring you the transformation you long for.
- You love exercise, but struggle with time – getting to a gym three times per week just isn't always possible.
- You like the idea of making your walk to work a highly effective workout without the blood, sweat and tears.

If you identify with any of the above, you're ready to embark on Walkactive and I'd love you to join me.

WHY YOU WALK WRONG

We're going to start by unpicking exactly what is going wrong with the way you are walking now. To do this, it's important to understand a bit about how your body works.

How your muscles work

When a muscle contracts (squeezes) it can create movement in several ways – the most common being when it shortens. Imagine holding a weight in one hand and doing a simple bicep curl: you need to bend at the elbow in order to bring the weight up and, as your hand moves towards your shoulder, the muscle fibres in your bicep get shorter – both ends of the muscle, where they are attached to the bone, move closer together. When we exercise in traditional ways such as jogging or lifting weights we tend to use this contracting movement again and again.

However, many people don't realise that it is possible for a muscle to carry on working hard as it lengthens back down too. Imagine a drawbridge: it doesn't just come crashing down, it is lowered in a controlled way. It's the same with Walkactive. Let's go back to that bicep curl again; this time, imagine lowering the same weight slowly, with control – don't just let that hand flop down. This takes effort, doesn't it? Your muscle is getting longer again, but as it lengthens, it is still working hard. In fact, the fibres in the muscle are still contracting, even though the muscle is getting longer. Because it takes effort, this lengthening movement tones the muscle. And with Walkactive this is happening all the time. Unlike most forms of exercise, such as running, where your muscles are primarily trying to contract, or shorten, most of the time, with Walkactive, we are trying to keep your muscles lenghtened as they contract, creating tone and greater strength and range of motion around the joint.

By doing this again and again, your muscles, quite literally, elongate. And this is why, with Walkactive, you can transform your entire appearance: you'll become taller, leaner, more streamlined and more poised.

Lifestyle and bad habits

Many of us spend hours every day hunched over computer screens, slumped in the car or in front of the TV. When we do move we may be carrying heavy bags or children or talking on a mobile phone – often all three at once. To cope with these unreasonable demands and stresses our bodies begin to use the wrong muscles at the wrong time and in the wrong way. Most people have already developed bad walking habits without even realising it, and these habits cause long-term pain and discomfort. They also stop us from using our muscles to their full potential as we walk.

Exercise

It is also possible that your existing regime is making your muscles even shorter. If you are already making the effort to keep fit, then the chances are that you choose exercise such as running, playing sport or working out at the gym. These kinds of exercise use your big muscle groups – those in your legs, bottom and torso, and while this can burn off a lot of calories and improve your fitness, it can also make your body's problem worse. Working only the large muscle groups will:

- thicken muscles rather than streamlining them – you are strengthening and shortening the big muscles in your body at the same time and this gives you a bulky rather than elegant, streamlined silhouette
- cause discomfort in your thoracic spine, neck and joints – specifically your hips, knees, shoulders – as the imbalance created by your shortened muscles puts them under strain
- cause even more postural problems because as you focus on the big muscles, the deeper, internal supportive muscles – those that are essential for good posture – are hardly stimulated at all; again, this makes your structural alignment even worse, putting your body out of balance and causing all sorts of injuries, aches and pains.

THE MECHANICS OF WALKING WRONG

So we've seen what contributes to walking wrong. But what, from a technical point of view, makes this happen? There are four key elements to walking wrong and I'm going to take you through them now, starting with your feet and ankles, moving on to your big leg muscles, then your head, neck and upper back and finally your arms and shoulders.

1. Your feet and ankles

Problem: the passive foot strike

A passive foot strike is one of the most common walk-wrong problems. Your foot and ankle have three 'rockers' (pivot points): the heel, the ball of the foot and the toes – see below. These should work together to create a smooth 'rolling' movement: from the heel, to the ball of the foot, to the toes. But for most of us, this important rolling or rocking movement has been lost, and the foot hits the ground more or less flat, all in one go.

The impact of this travels all the way up your body, from your feet through your knees and hips. This puts stress on your joints and can compress the discs in your spine (this is one reason why many people get knee, hip and back pain as they age). It also stops the muscles in your foot and your lower leg from moving as well as they should. Over time, your foot becomes less and less mobile or pliable – and it no longer sends the same feedback to your brain. This lack of feedback, in turn, affects your balance, posture and the quality of your movements. You grow increasingly unsteady and begin to move with a more 'shuffling' gait – your feet going straight down, rather than rolling and springing. Your foot's muscle tone becomes poor and weak, you are more likely to injure and strain yourself and you lose – quite literally – the 'spring in your step'. This feedback from foot to brain is called proprioception. It is a vital part of Walkactive.

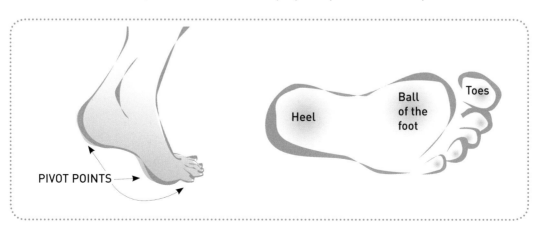

PIVOT POINTS

Heel   Ball of the foot   Toes

2. Your big leg muscles

Problem: tight muscles that work too hard

The big muscles on the front and the top half of your leg form one of the strongest muscle groups in the human body. The simplest way for you to move your leg forward is to use these muscles – so you use them all the time. However, since you also sit down a lot, these strong muscles grow used to being in a shortened position. This shortening curtails your range of movement, and throws off the alignment of the spine, directly contributing to lower-back pain. It is an unfortunate – yet extremely common – chain reaction. The big leg muscles are overused at the expense of the muscles in your bottom and down the back of your legs – these muscles are brilliant at burning up calories, and are vital for the shape and tone of the lower body. In the course of this book,

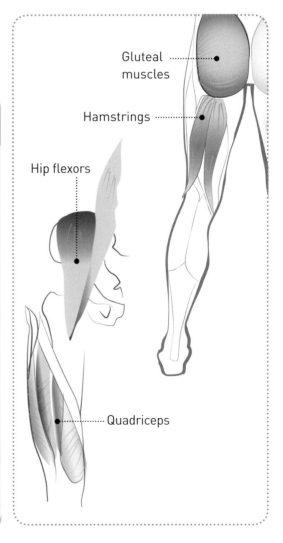

Gluteal muscles

Hamstrings

Hip flexors

Quadriceps

Leg Muscles: the Technical Bits

The long muscles that run up the front of your thigh from your kneecap, threading through your pelvis to attach to your lumbar spine, are known as the hip flexors. If you've ever walked a longer distance than usual and noticed that your lower back aches, this will be due to tight hip flexors.

The large muscles that run from the top of your thigh to your knee are your quadriceps (or 'quads'). If you are a sports player, your quads will be strong as these are the main muscles that drive forward.

The muscles in your bottom are your gluteal muscles (or 'glutes') and those down the back of your legs are your hamstrings. If you aren't using your glutes and hamstrings as much as you could then, apart from any structural problems you are causing, you're missing a trick! You are bypassing some serious toning, posture-enhancing and calorie-burning opportunities.

Neck and Upper Back: the Technical Bits

The bone and muscles of your upper back between your shoulder blades are known as the thoracic spine. Many people are tight and immobile here because they are walking wrong – and their posture is bad. This immobility causes the neck muscles (the sternacleidomastoid muscles) to grow tight and short, making the problem worse. The human body is designed to work as a unit - so when your upper body becomes stiff, there is a direct knock-on effect on the rest of your body. If your shoulders become stiff and their range of movement is restricted, this will restrict the movement in your lower back and hips.

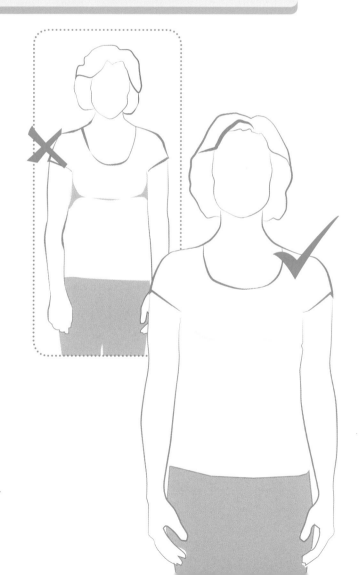

you'll learn how to change your habits to use all these muscles correctly, so your body becomes balanced, toned and elongated, while burning off more calories.

3. Your head, neck and upper back

Problem: limited movement and asymmetry Our modern lifestyles wreak havoc on this area of the body. All those hours hunched in the wrong posture, or carrying objects and children in the wrong way, lead to stiff shoulders and back. And this makes your shoulders slump forward (see right) and your spine stiffen – a major cause of back pain. The result is a clunky way of moving, not to mention a lot of pain and discomfort. The shoulders should be relaxed and down.

4. Your arms and shoulders

Problem: poor shoulder alignment and reduced natural arm swing If your shoulders and mid-back are not as mobile as they should be, then your arms will not swing naturally to and fro as you walk. Again, this has a surprising impact on your whole spine. The spine should rotate gently as you walk (see right), but if your arms are not swinging correctly then your spine is not rotating, and you are not fully using the muscles along the sides of your body either (your oblique muscles, see diagram below). So whether you are a man or a woman, your stiff arms and shoulders are unwittingly standing between you and the svelte shape you want to be!

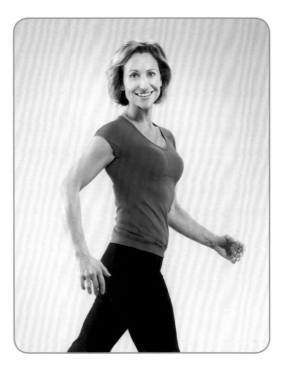

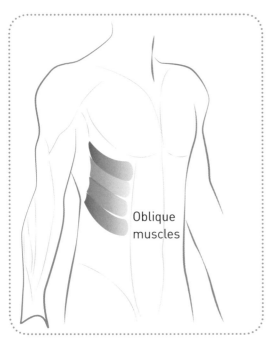

Oblique muscles

'I'm very overweight, so when I attended Joanna's Walkactive Spa Break I felt a little nervous at first. I've tried so many things, and so often I've ended up with pain in my knees and back. But I thought I'd give this a go. After ninety minutes of Walkactive – probably the most activity I've done in a good four or five years – I woke up the next day pain-free. I was amazed! This was the first time I'd woken up without any back pain or discomfort in two years. I realised then that this really does work. I now walk every day and feel so much better. Joanna's method has totally changed the way my body feels.'

TINA, 45, ATTENDED WALKACTIVE SPA BREAK

Why Walkactive is Better for You Than Power Walking

Walkactive is never to be confused with power walking. Power walking – that fast, wiggling, robotically-stiff walk – may seem like a good fitness strategy: you think you are reducing your joint impact because you're not running. You also have your body tense and your bottom and abs clenched, for maximum toning benefit. But, in fact, this forces you to use your muscles in completely the wrong way. It can cause injury and it will not bring you the body you want. With power walking, your hip flexors power you forward and you pull in your glutes and stomach muscles (abdominals or 'abs') in an attempt to tone hips, thighs and bottom, but this tightening movement limits the length of your strides, and to cope with the unnatural small-stepped movement, your lower back braces itself. This causes all sorts of lower-back problems and also stops you from using your abs as much as you could. You therefore get neither the tummy nor the bottom-toning effect you'd hoped for when you power walk. Instead you get back strain. My advice on power walking is simple: don't do it!

HOW TO WALK RIGHT

So we've looked at what is wrong with the way you walk. Now it's time to fix these problems and learn how to walk right.

The Walkactive system will teach you to:

- **unravel the wrong movement pattern** – you learn to identify what you're doing wrong and switch off those wrong muscle groups
- **create the correct movement pattern** – you learn to switch on the correct muscle groups, using them in the right way and at the right time – I call this 're-ravelling'
- **embed your technique** – you practise so that your new correct movement

pattern becomes second nature; you'll notice that the new movements you've learned feel more fluid and relaxed, and you'll notice the results too (toned muscles, inch loss, increased fitness, among others).

Walkactive is a process of reconnecting with your body, so you may find you have to really concentrate as you learn how to walk right. You are recruiting muscles that have grown very used to sitting on the sidelines while others do the work. At first, those muscles will be reluctant to work. They might even object, loudly, to being asked to participate. But keep asking them to cooperate, and they will. Ultimately, your body will love you for this.

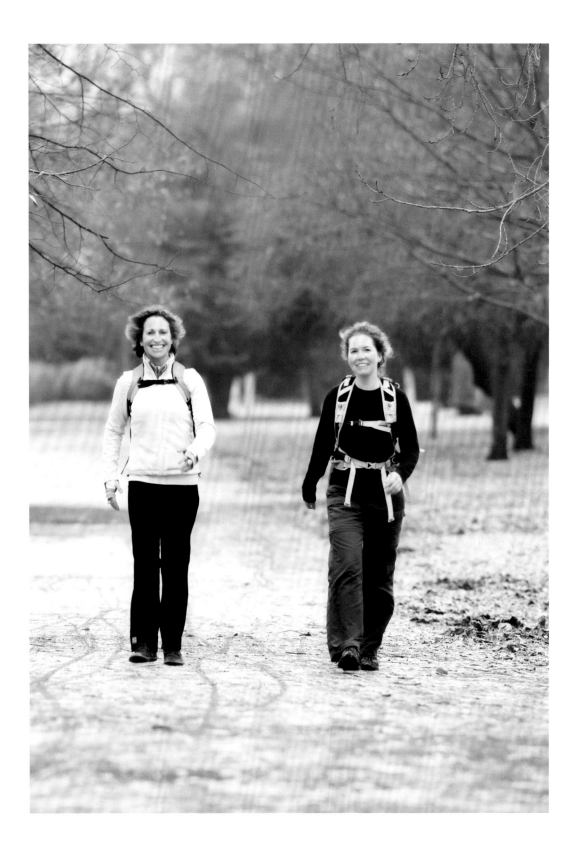

'By learning Walkactive, I feel I'm understanding the amazing things my body can do without artificial enhancements or strain. I walk taller and feel far more elegant. Walkactive is, quite simply, helping me to be the most real and beautiful woman I can possibly be – naturally.'

PIPPA, 35, JOINED A WALKACTIVE CLUB

Walkactive will ensure you...

Use the right muscles

Walkactive teaches you to use the muscles in the front of your legs less and those at the back of your leg and bottom more.

Result: improved muscle tone all over your body and more effective fat burning.

Use your muscles in the right way

Walkactive teaches you to minimise the movements (muscle contractions) that make your muscles grow shorter. Instead you learn how to contract your muscles *as they lengthen.*

Result: your muscles become leaner, longer and more taut.

Use your muscles at the right time

Contracting all your muscles at the same time as you exercise creates tension, compresses some parts of the body and limits your range of motion. Walkactive teaches you how to contract your muscles at the right time – relaxing them before they contract again.

Result: a smooth and fluid way of moving that does not put pressure or strain on joints.

Use your muscles in the right sequence

The last piece in the Walkactive jigsaw is learning to contract your muscles in the right sequence.

Result: when your muscles move in the correct sequence you walk in a smooth, fluid way, with the correct postural alignment, using your muscles to their full potential – you will feel like you are gliding.

To achieve these objectives, we're going to focus on four key Walkactive body parts. If you master these, you will walk right. They are:

- your feet and ankles
- your hips
- your neck and upper back
- your arms and shoulders.

'I've had so many pains in my muscles and joints (I have polymyalgia rheumatica) and I often still wake up with some stiffness and aches. But Walkactive has definitely loosened up all these joints and muscles so much. Now, after walking, I feel so much better than before. Best of all, I can incorporate Walkactive into my everyday life. I am now so aware of how I'm walking (wherever I'm walking – even down to the shops). This has been an amazing thing for my body – I really can feel the intelligent exercise working on me from the inside out!'

JULIE, 50, ATTENDED WALKACTIVE WALK FIRM COURSE

So all this might sound a bit technical and complicated. But don't worry – absolutely anyone can learn Walkactive and I'll be guiding you throughout each stage, so that it will all make sense to you. I also use a 'skill-layering' approach, whereby I teach you how to master one body part at a time. Then, when you're ready, you put all four body parts together and hey presto – that's Walkactive!

WHY WALKACTIVE IS 'INTELLIGENT EXERCISE'

I call Walkactive 'intelligent exercise' because it realigns your body from the inside out. Intelligent exercise:

- creates space between the joints, so you can achieve correct postural alignment, so you feel and look amazing and energetic – and you lose the aches and pains

- helps the deep internal muscles to support the joints: your joints can at last move freely, the way they are meant to move, no longer limited and restricted, robbing you of your height, good posture and range of motion

- builds a strong internal framework, beginning with your bones and working outwards, through the supportive muscles; your big muscles will then 'shrink-wrap' themselves around this taut, lean framework (instead of bulking up and pulling your body out of alignment).

IS WALKING ENOUGH?

Most people assume that they have to do something really vigorous such as jogging or a gym class for an hour three times per week, if they want to see results. They start regimes with the best intentions, but then real life kicks in – social events, family

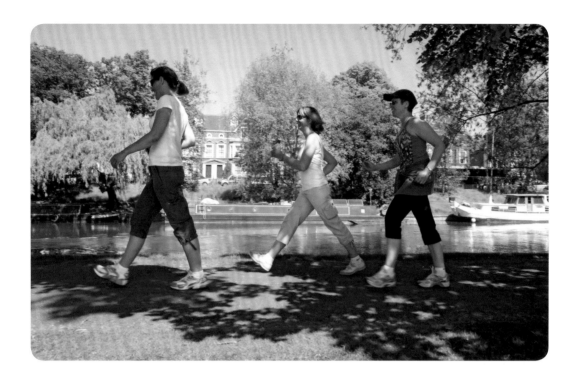

commitments, long hours at work, endless chores, dark nights closing in and so on. And things tend to slip. Before they know it, their amazing new regime is 'broken' and they are back into their old, bad habits again. They feel like they've failed.

If this sounds familiar to you, I'm not surprised. But it's not going to happen again. Walkactive is different. It is not a 'regime' – it's a way of life. It is about changing your habits in a very manageable way, so that you never want to go back. Walkactive can bring you all the body benefits of a strong workout – and more – with none of the pain, boredom or enforced routines.

Why Walkactive is better than running

Walking 'wrong' and running burn roughly the same number of calories over the same distance and at similar speeds. If you run faster than you walk, you will burn more calories, but you may not get the toning benefits you hope for. Many women take up jogging in order to change their shape. They think it will bring streamlined thighs and hips. However, when you jog you are not contracting your glutes (bottom muscles) properly. Walkactive may be slower than running, but it tones your body much more effectively because it uses all your muscles in the right way.

Walking and running also affect your joints and muscles in different ways. Let's take a look in more detail at why, exactly, Walkactive is more effective – and better for your body – than running.

1. Your knee angle, muscles and joints

Your knees bend more in a running stride than they do in a walking stride. This means that your foot hits the ground with more force when you run than when you walk, and the greater impact puts more stress on your joints. This increased knee bend, as you run, also uses your quads (front thigh muscles) more than walking does. This is one reason why, when you run, your knees and quad muscles become more tired than they do when you walk the same distance. This running knee movement contracts – and tightens – the quads and hip flexors, but it does not work the glutes and hamstrings to the same extent. All of this will strain your posture and muscle tone, as explained earlier (see page 16).

2. Speed and joint impact

Running speeds vary widely from runner to runner, but in general, the faster you run, the more impact the movement has on your joints. With Walkactive, however, the impact on your joints does not increase the faster you go. In fact, your movements remain fluid and

healthy with Walkactive regardless of how fast you go. Most people can, of course, run faster than they can walk. But with Walkactive, your pace will speed up a lot as you adjust your technique. The big difference is that unlike jogging, you can increase your pace without increasing joint impact or strain.

'As I got older, I realised running is just not for me – so I'm a walker now, and I love it. But with Walkactive, I noticed a significant increase in my pace even after just one session. I felt much lighter and faster without having to force my speed. I didn't realise walking could be this effective. Walkactive has taken walking to a whole new level for me and my body.'
ANNA, 48, AFTER JUST ONE FIFTY-MINUTE WALKACTIVE SESSION

3. Ground contact

Another significant difference between running and walking is the length of time your feet are in contact with the ground. When you walk, at least one of your feet is in contact with the ground at any given time. The same is not true of running, where both your feet can be off the ground at the same time. When you walk, your foot is in contact with the ground for longer than when you run. With Walkactive the contact between foot and the ground is even more important because you roll through your foot and push

CASE STUDY: JEREMY – PERSISTENCE PAYS OFF

Jeremy had noticed the weight creeping on, but with long hours at work he didn't have time for the gym. He had always discounted walking as being a 'girly' activity that would never really give him the results he'd want, especially since he walked during his daily commute and hadn't noticed any change to his body shape or fitness. So when his girlfriend told him she was going on a 'walking course', he was dubious.

'I wondered what Joanna could possibly teach her about walking that she hadn't already grasped over the previous thirty-six years!' he says. 'But somehow, I ended up being roped in. On day one Joanna explained the science behind her technique and walked us through the implementation. While I wouldn't admit it, I could feel my posture changing right there. Between then and my second session, my girlfriend also commented on how my feet seemed to have been silenced as they touched the floor. I went to the second session and this time I felt my muscles starting to really work. After the walk I felt as though I'd been to the gym.

'The technique is hard to master at first. It's not something you can pick up in one session; it needs to be practised for your body to adjust to this new way of walking. But it felt good, so I kept going, and after four weeks I was amazed to find that I'd lost five inches [12.5 cm] in body mass. Men tend to have preconceptions that walking is for girls. But Joanna's Walkactive technique makes total sense for my body – it works for weight management and it's actually very enjoyable so you can easily integrate it into your daily life. It's become part of my life now!'

'After four weeks I was amazed to find that I'd lost five inches [12.5 cm] in body mass. Men tend to have preconceptions that walking is for girls. But Joanna's Walkactive technique makes total sense for my body'

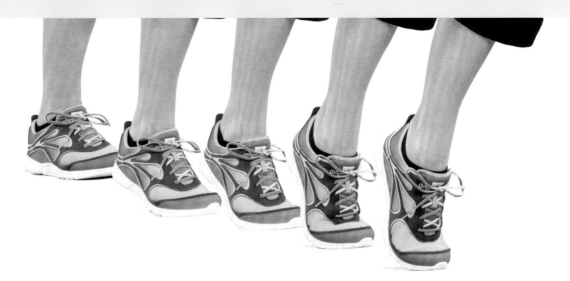

off the ground with your toes (see above). This movement gives you amazing shaping and toning results in your bottom and legs, and these muscles also burn more calories, so it is great for weight loss. So Walkactive is more effective than jogging because the rolling, powering movement of your foot and ankle against the ground uses the muscles in your bottom far more than running can.

'I love what Walkactive does to my body. I've always loved running, but after my physio and my masseuse told me that running was creating all sorts of problems for my body, I reluctantly gave it up. That's when I tried Walkactive. My physio and masseuse tell me that my body is in better shape than it's ever been. I'm lighter and more taut and my posture is so much better. I'll never go back to running now.'

SARAH, 57, WALKACTIVE BESPOKE CLIENT

In the next chapter, I'm going to teach you the basic Walkactive techniques. Every step you take can be one towards transformation, whatever your age, phase or stage of life. Whether you're in your twenties, thirties, forties, fifties, sixties, seventies, eighties or nineties – it works the same way.

If all of this sounds too good to be true and you are feeling a little sceptical – well, I understand. But give it a go. You've got nothing to lose. Walkactive is about applying science to the way your body should and can move. I have studied exercise physiology in great detail for years, and I know that if you follow my instructions, you'll achieve the outcome you want. I promise.

So as you move on to the next chapter, here's what I want you to do:

1. **Follow the process in the order I tell you**
Mastering Walkactive is sequential: each body part's actions have a direct knock-on effect on the next.

2. **Take it slow** Trust your body and trust my experience. I've taught Walkactive to hundreds of people and I've seen again and again what it can do – and how much people love it. I want you to enjoy the process of connecting with your body. If you rush it, it's harder to actually enjoy, and the results are more difficult to achieve. As I often tell clients: *life is hard if you take it by the yard – but life is a cinch if you take it by the inch!*

3. **Focus on the process not the outcome**
The outcome is a better posture, inches off your waistline, a longer, more relaxed stride and countless other long-term health benefits. But don't get hung up on all this. Just apply the process and the outcome will take care of itself.

4. **Accept a bit of frustration** We live in a fast-paced world, where we are promised instant success – now! Now! Now! I'm not going to mislead you – Walkactive will take time to master. But once you do master it, you'll see improvements in a very short time.

'I started a Walkactive course and within four weeks, I had lost 5 inches [12.5cm] off my waistline and hips and, most surprisingly, I had actually gained an inch [2.5cm] in height – not bad for someone of sixty-seven. I was amazed!'

SUE, ATTENDED TWENTY-EIGHT-DAY WALK OFF WEIGHT COURSE

Sue is just one of thousands of people who have transformed their bodies and lives with Walkactive. But don't just take my word for it – try it for yourself. Start connecting, right here, right now, with the way your body should move, can move and will move. You'll be so glad you did.

CHAPTER TWO

MASTERING WALKACTIVE

'I used to go running and I'd come home feeling strung out and sort of "jolted", then there'd be aches and pains. After Walkactive I feel relaxed and my body feels stretched, but not strained. I'm fitter than I was when I was running too. It's an addictive feeling.'

OK, so now it's time to get to grips with the basics of the Walkactive technique. I'm going to teach you to walk so you tone up your muscles, burn more calories and feel and look completely amazing. You're going to reconnect with your body so that it moves smoothly, fluidly, correctly and effectively. To do this, we're going to disconnect you from the wrong movements, and establish the correct movement patterns in their place. But I'm going to be honest with you here: on your first time out, this won't feel completely natural – or easy.

You won't feel you've mastered Walkactive when you've finished putting all the tips and advice in this chapter into your body for the first time. What you will feel, however, is:

- an improvement in your posture
- a change to your pace
- a positive difference in the way your body is moving.

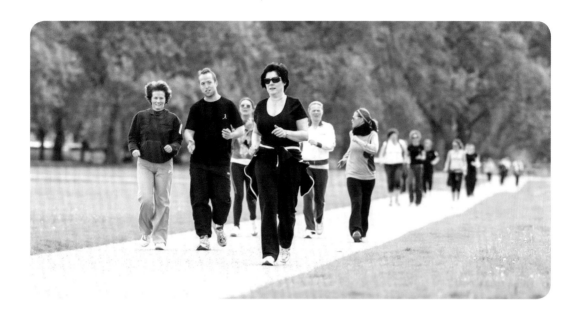

The key to getting results lies in the detail – it is vital to get the technique right. And this takes practice – lots of practice. But this doesn't mean you have to set aside hours of walking time. In fact, it is best to do your Walkactive practice sessions in really small chunks at first: as short as ten or fifteen minutes at a time, with each session focusing on one body part – the 'skill-layering' approach I mentioned in the previous chapter.

I'm asking you to start like this because it is easy to overload your brain and body when you're learning a whole new way of walking. And when your brain gets overloaded, your technique goes out the window. So try to be patient and don't rush it. I want you to trust my years of experience, my Walkactive process and, most of all, your own body. This will work if you do it right – but to do it right, you have to take it slow.

Now, I can't wait to get you started, so let's begin!

WHAT KIT DO I NEED?

The beauty of Walkactive is that you don't need much 'kit'. At first, it is important to focus on technique rather than how fast you go, so you won't even get particularly hot or sweaty. You just need a simple pedometer to count your steps, basic comfortable clothes and some flat shoes – ideally ones that allow your foot to spread, and that don't have too rigid a sole. (I talk more about kit in Chapter Four: Just Do It, pages 73 and 87–90.)

READY, STEADY, WALK!

So let's now take a look at exactly what it is you need to do.

Technique Walks

I want you to block out ten or fifteen minutes, ideally three times per day, every day. During these sessions, you are going to practise working on each of the four body parts discussed in the previous chapter, one at a time, until you've mastered all of them. I call these sessions your Technique Walks. To master Walkactive it's absolutely vital to set aside some time purely to focus on your technique. Of course, how fast you master each of the individual Walkactive body parts will depend on how often you practise, but there are other factors too, such as your fitness or your connection to your body. The bottom line is that you should keep doing your Technique Walks until you feel you've really got it.

To start your Technique Walks, all you need to do is put on a pair of flat, trainer-style flexible shoes and go outside. Ideally, you want to be on a flat-ish surface – the park or a level pavement is best. You start with your feet and, when you feel you've mastered your Walkactive feet – and that could take several Technique Walks – only then should you move on to your hips, and so on. Try not to rush too quickly from one body part to the

Not Just Simple Addition

Maths was not my best subject at school, but I like to think that mastering the four parts of Walkactive isn't just about making your walk four times better. As you master each body part (the feet, hips, neck and shoulders and arms), you multiply the benefits to the others you have already learned. And the more time you take over improving each part, the greater the benefit will be to the rest of your body, not to mention your mind, heart and soul. In other words, with Walkactive, the sum of the parts is greater than the whole. Learning to walk this way is deeply rewarding, whatever stage of life you're at. And it can be rather addictive.

FEET **X** HIPS **X** NECK & SHOULDERS **X** ARMS = **WALKACTIVE** next. It's really tempting, but it won't work in your favour. At the very least, focus on one body part per day. The more time you take to perfect and connect with each stage of the process, the more benefits you'll see.

Finally, don't be tempted to skip these Technique Walks altogether, and just bung it all together. If you do, you'll never see the true Walkactive benefits, because you'll never get it right. Take your time – and have fun with it.

Let's look at exactly what you are aiming for with each body part.

Technique 1: your feet

Aim: to stop passive foot strike (see below) and achieve an active foot and open ankle.

Payoff: improves balance; kick-starts correct alignment into the knee and so helps to protect your joints; jump-starts your body-shape change as you start using the correct muscles.

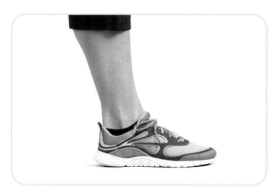

How to do it

At this point you should try not to worry about anything other than *how* your feet are moving, as follows:

Be aware of the various foot parts: as you start to put one foot in front of the other notice each of your feet's component parts. Every time you put a foot down, observe your heel, foot arch, ball of the foot and the toes. Each part has an important role to play.

Roll the foot: keep rolling through each foot as you walk, in a fluid action. Feel how your foot starts to become more 'active' than 'passive'. When your foot is passive, it hits the ground in one go as a single unit. When it's active, the different parts touch down as you roll through from heel to toe.

Soften the foot: think of your foot becoming more pliable as you gently roll through it. Imagine it is made of plasticine that has been left on a windowsill all day in the sun. If you picked it up it would be soft and pliable and you could mould it easily in your hand.

Spread the foot: you might feel that the ball of your foot wants to spread inside your shoe – this is good! Start to appreciate the *breadth* of your foot. If your shoes are a little tight-fitting, you may feel restricted here,

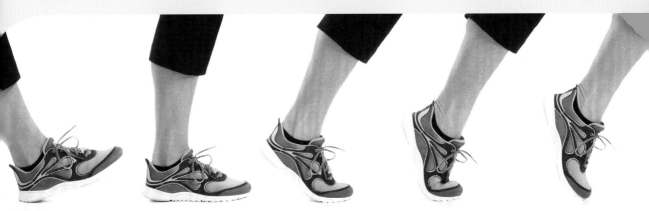

Achieving an 'open' ankle

but as your foot begins to spread, keep it soft and see if you can focus on propelling your body forward. Think of your body as a canoe: if you want the canoe to travel forward you pull the paddle past your body, then push the water behind you. As you do so, the canoe (your body) moves forward. Think of your feet as the paddles moving you smoothly forward.

Aim for active toes: now see if you can become aware of your big, middle and little toes. Start to feel these three areas with each step. As your foot is rolling forward, think of pushing evenly off your big toe, middle toe and little toe. (See 'Why your toes matter', opposite.)

Be aware of your heel strike: as your body starts to get used to this new way of walking, you'll see that the contact point between your heel and the ground is changing too. If you notice that your heel touches down on the pad rather than the edge, this is good! It helps to minimise the impact on your joints, as you have more cushioning on the pad of the heel and the impact is distributed over a greater surface area than if your heel hits the ground on its rim.

Aim for 'open' ankles: as your foot starts to become more active, you'll begin to notice that your ankle joint moves more too – you'll start to feel the front of your ankle opening up as you roll through your foot (as above). This 'open' ankle is a really important part of your technique. It will help to lengthen your leg muscles, streamline your thighs and kick-start the contraction of the muscles in your bottom. Make sure you don't bring your foot off the floor in a rush. Peeling your foot (see right) off the ground slowly helps to achieve an open ankle and stops you from rushing. So make this your mantra: *feel the peel!*

Why your toes matter

Feeling each of the big, middle and little toes (as described earlier) will help your foot to touch the ground evenly. This encourages correct alignment all the way up through your foot, knee and hips, which, in turn, helps you to engage the correct muscles in your bottom and the backs of your thighs. This doesn't just tone you up, transforming the way you look, it also helps your knee joints to stay healthy by keeping your knees aligned correctly. Isn't it amazing what toes can do?

'When I started Walkactive I found it quite easy to get an active foot, but getting the open ankle was harder. However, when I started to feel my ankles open up more, I noticed that the muscles in my whole leg started to feel like they were lengthening too. This also improved my pace – and then I began to feel my bottom muscles working more too! I couldn't believe that all this could come from one little ankle!'

MEROPE, 35, AFTER A BESPOKE WALKACTIVE SESSION

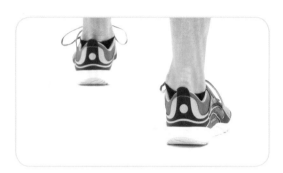

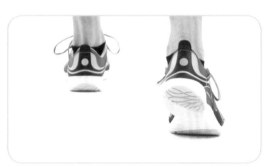

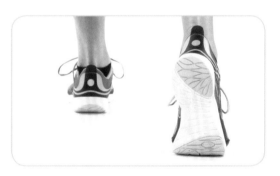

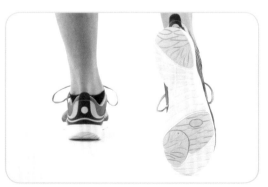

Peeling the foot

TIP *Compare your feet and hands*

If you are struggling to get any movement into your feet, open up your hand and look at it as you pretend to knead that piece of warm plasticine (see page 31). Watch how much your hand can move – your wrist, knuckles, the bones and joints along each of your fingers. Although the digits are shorter on the feet, the bone arrangement is the same as in the hands. This means that our feet could have a similar range and degree of movement as our hands, but we have lost this ability to move because we don't use our feet properly. But if you make your toes active (see below), you'll get a lot of movement and strength back, and you'll notice a huge difference in your feet, and in the rest of your body too. Don't worry – it will come with practice.

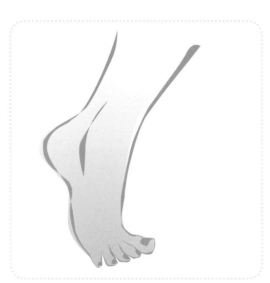

'At first it was difficult to get any flexibility in my feet at all – they were so used to being immobile and they constantly hit the ground as one unit. But within a week's practice of Walkactive I noticed that my feet were a lot more mobile, and felt much less stiff. I also noticed that the skin on my feet got softer as I started to use my feet more effectively.'
KAREN, 48, ATTENDED WALKACTIVE INTRODUCTORY WORKSHOP

Feel the rhythm
As you roll fluidly through the heel, arch, breadth of your foot and toes – giving a gentle push forward as you come through the foot – try to get into a rhythm. Don't rush your peeling feet; enjoy this natural rhythm. And as you get into it, you'll soon feel how your feet are moving differently, and your momentum will change – you'll feel as if you are moving forward more easily, and at a quicker pace.

TROUBLESHOOTING
'It feels bouncy!' If at this stage you feel you are bouncing with each step, rather than floating forward, don't worry – it means you are on your way to an active foot. When you start out, the transition from a passive to an active foot and open ankle is a big one. The bouncy movement happens because you are

propelling yourself forward by pushing off the ball of your foot instead of rolling from the ball to the junction between the ball and your toes, opening your ankles, and then pushing off your toes. So stick at it! As your ankles and feet begin to move more, you'll flex and roll more easily, and this bounce will evolve into a confident, lean stride.

'I've got claw feet'

As you concentrate hard to master the correct movement pattern – through your brain–muscle pathway (see page 43) – it's common to tense up the feet, creating a claw-like foot. This can cause the front of your feet to feel achy and painful and can make it difficult to get that soft, rolling movement. So try to think of your feet as soft and pliable. It can help to imagine that there is Velcro on the floor and on the bottom of your shoes – with each step you are peeling your relaxed foot off the Velcro.

Technique 2: your hips

Aim: to stop slumping into your hips (see far right); to achieve hip stability without rigidity; to start to feel a hip lift (see right).

Payoff: you'll continue improving your knee and hip alignment and this will reduce the impact on your joints; you'll start to tighten your lower abdominal muscles, trimming your torso; your bottom will start to lift,

tighten and work properly; if you have back problems, your pain will be minimised; you'll notice that you can go faster.

How to do it

Imagine glasses of water on your hips: try to envisage a tray extending out from your hip bones, with two glasses of water on it. As you walk, try to lift up and out of your hips so that the glasses of water are also lifted up evenly, but remain full. If you pull your stomach in too tight and start to clench your bottom, then your pelvis will tilt too far and those glasses of water will spill. If your imaginary glasses of water start to spill, it means your posture is wrong. If it helps to motivate you, try imagining the glasses contain not water, but your favourite tipple!

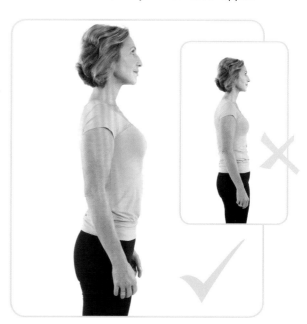

Abdominal J: now you need to focus on your abdominal muscles as you lift and stabilise those hips. As you walk forward, lifting your hips and keeping the imaginary tray steady, try to draw your stomach *in and also, very importantly, up*. This is not the same as simply sucking your tummy in (see 'The Abdominal J' box opposite – you are trying to achieve the same but without holding the contraction). As you perform this inward and upward movement, you should feel as if your spine has grown a little taller.

'After five days with Joanna tweaking my technique and encouraging me on my Abdominal Js my waistline is 2 inches (5cm) smaller, trimmer, neater. I was not the best person in the group at the technique by a long way, and certainly not the fittest or most naturally sporty, but I was seriously impressed with how the Abdominal Js trimmed my waistline!'
ZARA, 40, ATTENDED WALKACTIVE INTERNATIONAL TRAINING CAMP

Why your hips matter

If you are tilting your pelvis, you won't get the maximum Walkactive benefits because the muscles in your bottom won't contract correctly. This will slow you down, and stop you getting the body transformation you want. If you are also used to sucking in your abs in an attempt to tone your tummy, while simultaneously tightening your bottom, then this is a big mistake: it compresses your lower back and can cause back pain. Hip stability without rigidity on the other hand, perks up your derrière, reduces back discomfort and flattens and trims your torso. So keep those hips stable and those water glasses full.

TROUBLESHOOTING

'I can't feel the right muscles.' The hip lift can be tricky, so don't panic if you are finding this hard. But you can do it. To do it properly you have to connect with and use deep internal muscles which may not have been used for quite a while, but you will eventually find them, and they will really help to transform your body. Try to think about standing up as tall as possible, but imagine that the height you achieve does not just come from lifting up out of your waistline and stretching up through your spine – rather, it starts at your knees. You are pulling everything upwards from there, up through the front of the legs, towards your hips. It may take a while to feel this movement, but keep trying.

'My back aches!' If you start to feel discomfort in your back, the chances are you are pulling in through your abs too much. This is quite common. It is important to think of lifting your abdominals in and up – in that J shape – rather than just pulling them in tight and back towards your spine, which encourages

The Abdominal J

This is my number-one, all-round best abdominal exercise. Get it right and it works miracles. It is also the perfect way to help you master your hip lift (hip stability without rigidity – see page 35).

- Stand with good posture and your weight distributed evenly on both feet. Visualise a capital letter J in front of you. The long part of the J is closest to your body and the short part is furthest away.

- In your mind, imagine you are tracing over the J with your abdominals. So starting at the bottom by your pubic bone, 'scoop' out your abs and then draw them in and up towards your sternum, as if drawing up the long part of the letter J (see sequence below). Don't worry about the cross at the top of the 'J' – just imagine your J as a curve. The long part of the J is you drawing upward.

- To help you imagine this, slide your fingertips between your waistband and your tummy. Pull your tummy muscles in and up at the same time – away from your fingers – without expanding your ribcage or tensing your back muscles. Don't take deep breaths or hold your breath.

- Hold this contraction for a count of ten, then relax for ten. Repeat five to ten times.

- Make sure your ribcage is down – your chest should not be 'puffed up'. Your ribs should taper down not out and your bottom should be relaxed, your back lengthened, not contracted.

As you do this, you are lengthening the area between your pubic bone and your breast bone – imagine these two points moving further apart: your abdominal muscles are getting longer, leaner and flatter as you do this lengthening movement. The upward lengthening movement of the J tones your abdominal area far more effectively than just sucking in your tummy. Do it as often as you can and you'll see a huge difference: a flat abdomen and fabulous inch loss.

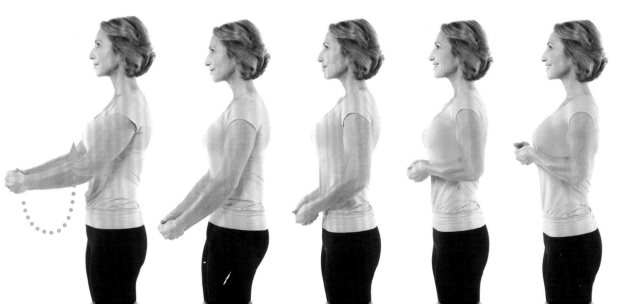

Understanding Your Hip Joint

Your hip joint is a ball-and-socket arrangement. It should be able to move in a variety of directions: forward ('flexion'), backward ('extension') and to the side ('adduction and abduction'). It should also rotate in its socket. Unfortunately, because of poor posture and the amount of time we spend sitting in cars or at our desks, most of us get very tight in our hip joints. The hip flexors (see diagram on page 16) and the quads are also tight and too short, and this also reduces the range of hip motion. As a result, our hip joints become compressed which, in turn, limits how we use the muscles in our bottoms (glutes) and our abdominals, and affects our overall body tone, power, shape and posture. It's astonishing what one joint is responsible for.

your lower back to 'brace' itself against the pressure, and to lock in place. This puts pressure on the lower back – which is what you're feeling. It also stops you from using the right muscles properly, so really gets in the way of the Walkactive technique. If this is happening to you, then let go and relax your abs. Now, start to draw them in and up again in that J shape, this time paying more attention to the lift up than the sucking in. Remember, even if you can't feel it, visualise it – you will be encouraging the brain to send the correct message to the targeted muscles and they will respond.

'On the first day of Joanna's Training Camp, when she introduced the Abdominal Js, I really did not feel anything – I totally loved the idea, but there just seemed to be no response in that part of my body. I'm only forty, with no kids, but still it seemed elusive. But at some point on the second day I did feel a change, and by the third day I was really noticing the difference every time I did them. By day four, my torso and waistline were feeling much more nipped in, and I was more aware of that area of my body the whole time. Abdominal Js really do work!'

ROSIE, 40, ATTENDED WALKACTIVE INTERNATIONAL TRAINING CAMP

The Pelvic Girdle

The muscles in your bottom are also attached to your pelvis (the 'pelvic girdle'). When you have stable hips and an active foot you will notice that the muscles in your bottom start to work harder too. This is because all your deepest 'core' muscles – including those in your bottom (your gluteal muscles) – are working together to keep your pelvic girdle steady. This is why hip stability is vital: it tones you up, safeguards the hip joint and maintains correct posture. (It also makes you move faster – see page 54 for an explanation of hip stability and pace.)

Technique 3: your neck and shoulders

Aim: to achieve symmetry through the torso.

Payoff: combats poor posture, especially slumped shoulders and rounded back; reduces tension in the upper back and helps mobility of shoulders, upper back and neck; achieves length and softness through the neck and upper body without looking stiff and tense; opens and softens shoulders, helping you to achieve correct back alignment; starts to get your body in the right position to whittle your waist as you walk.

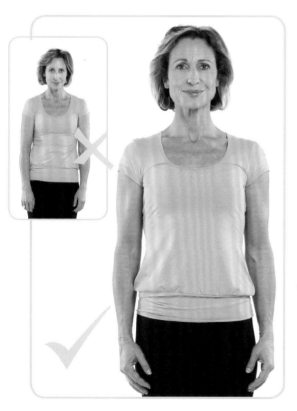

How to do it

- **Imagine dangly earrings**: keeping your feet active and your hips lifted, think about the distance between your ear lobes and shoulders. You're going to try and increase this distance. Imagine you have long, dangly earrings hanging from each ear lobe (or men might prefer to imagine two short rulers measuring the distance between their ear lobes and their shoulders). As you walk, you are trying to make sure the earrings or rulers don't touch your shoulders. Now imagine your shoulders gently falling away down your back (don't force them), and your neck gently lengthening. This opens your shoulders and chest area and encourages your spine to align itself correctly, right up through your body.

- **Try to relax**: Walkactive is about the body moving fluidly and smoothly. It shouldn't be stiff or tense. So rather than force these movements, try to 'allow' them to happen to your body. It's easy to tense up as you concentrate on getting it right, but if you catch yourself straining, try to let go.

- **Keep the rhythm**: remember to keep the rhythm of your walking going as you lengthen your neck and shoulders. There is a lot of activity and change happening in your body right now. Try to keep it smooth, rhythmic and relaxed.

Why your neck and shoulders matter

Getting your neck and shoulder positioning right has a huge knock-on effect on your body as a whole. It will improve your posture, and you'll instantly look better. It will also help to lengthen the muscles in this area, which can become very short from activities such as carrying bags or children and tapping away on a keyboard. This shortening causes the shoulders to roll and hunch, restricting their mobility as well as that of the upper back. This, in turn, limits the ability of your spine to rotate as you walk, thereby stopping the possible waist-whittling movement of every step you take.

Remember: keep taking it one body part at a time

The relationship between the hips and the neck and shoulders is interesting – in essence, I'm asking you to achieve a physical oxymoron: I want you to lift up out of your hips, while at the same time (eventually) relaxing down through your shoulders. This is why you need to take each body part separately at first: you are learning to layer in a skill with each technique. You might, for instance, focus on your hip lift in one session, then in another focus on your neck and shoulders. This way, you can perfect the movement without getting confused about which body part should be doing what. I will ask you to put them together – just not yet!

Technique 4: your arms

Aim: to achieve correct shoulder-girdle mobility; to get the arms to move like flowing pendulums as you walk.

Payoff: your back, neck and shoulders will start to love you as they become more agile; you'll enjoy better shape and tone in your chest and arms; you'll lay the foundations for significantly reducing back fat.

How to do it

By now you've mastered the feet, hips and neck and shoulders. You might already notice that your arms are swinging gently forward and backward with each step. If you have, then this is fantastic. This is how your body is meant to move – do let your arms move naturally, but add in these tweaks:

Imagine a pendulum: try to envisage each arm as a natural pendulum, moving forward and backward as you take each step.

Elbows: as your pendulum arms gently swing to and fro, I want you to introduce a slight bend at your elbow (see right). Try to focus on the backward movement, rather than the forward one – on drawing your elbow back and letting it swing naturally forward again. Don't keep your elbows low, 'pump' your arms or clench your fists. See if you can swing back further than you swing forward.

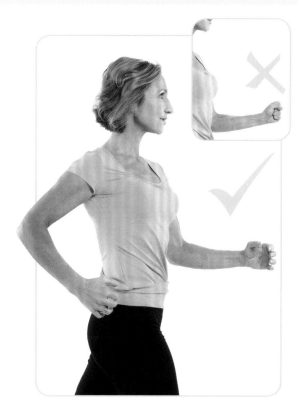

The more your elbows draw back like this, the more the front of your shoulders will open up. This correct arm movement will also improve your posture, giving you that instant energetic, slimmer, taller look.

Notice your swing: the shorter forward swing and longer, larger back swing described above will help to engage the shoulder girdle, putting vital mobility into your spine. As your arms swing, they should naturally move across towards the mid-line of the body. Your spine will start to rotate and the muscles that run up the sides of your torso (your oblique muscles) – will start to work too. This is a key

movement in Walkactive – it can literally take inches off your waistline because with every step your oblique muscles in your waist are working hard.

The short lever

When you start to move your arms, it is much easier to add a bend at the elbow so that your arms are shorter – in biomechanics we call this a 'short lever'. All it means is that it's easier for your body to control your arms if they are bent, rather than long, loose and flapping about. With a short lever it's easier to let the arm go back.

If your arms feel stiff, or you're worrying that having a bent elbow looks silly, don't worry – you're not going to be walking with stiff, bent elbows all the time. Your 'short lever' will help you get the hang of the arm movement as you start out, but as you get better at Walkactive the angle of the arm can open so that it's more of a 120-degree bend. Just make sure you maintain an awareness of the forearm (elbow to wrist).

TROUBLESHOOTING

'The arms don't feel right.' To help keep your arms relaxed, imagine that you are holding a crisp between your thumb and second finger: you have to hold your crisp without crushing it. This will help to keep the tension out of your hands and arms, which can stiffen your shoulder girdle and reduce the mobility of your upper back. Alternatively, imagine you are a dancer – a dancer's arm movements are very fluid and soft. It's the same with Walkactive. Try to appreciate the flow of the movement, rather than the rigidity.

 TIP ....
Lead with the elbows not the hands

Make sure you lead with the elbow – it should be the first thing that comes behind your body and not your hand (see below). If it is your hand, you'll be missing out on some serious waist-whittling benefits, as well as a fabulous shoulder mobilisation to ease a tight upper back.

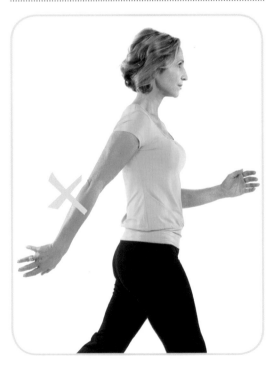

ALL TOGETHER NOW: PUTTING THE BODY PARTS TOGETHER

So if you have been practising each of the four body parts in your Technique Walks, one at a time in ten- or fifteen-minute slots, three times per day, this is what should be happening to you:

- Your feet are softer, pliable and more active – remember to keep pushing gently off your big, middle and little toes.
- Your hips are lifted – keep drawing up from the knees to the hips, making sure those glasses of water stay full with each step and creating your J shape with your abs.
- Your neck and shoulders are soft as you try to increase the distance between the ear lobes and your shoulders.
- You are naturally swinging your arms, with the emphasis more on backward movement and a bent elbow.

If all this is happening, then you're ready to put everything together and give it a go – you're ready to Walkactive! If it isn't happening, go back to basics: take one body part and just focus on it for a whole week – don't worry about anything else. Then, the next week, add another body part, so you are working on two parts together, and so on.

Brain-muscle Pathways

You're learning a whole new movement pattern and to do this you are creating what's known as a 'brain-muscle pathway'. You are unravelling old, incorrect movement patterns ('walking wrong') and creating new, correct ones, using the right muscles in the right way. This is complicated stuff and it takes practice. Your brain is working as hard as your body – this is why it can feel mentally challenging. So don't panic if your body feels stiff and awkward at first – this is quite normal. Your brain-muscle pathway is just establishing itself. It takes time.

You'll then get to grips with your technique over a four-week period.

Schedule your 'Give-it-a-go' sessions

Set aside two thirty- to forty-five-minute slots. These are your Give-it-a-go sessions, when you're going to put together everything you've learned about the four body parts. To do this, you need to get outside in flat shoes on a flat surface as usual, and take a watch or stopwatch with you. You're going to break your session up into approximately three- to five-minute slots and focus on adding in a body part at a time until your whole body is moving in Walkactive harmony.

Now give it a go and start walking!

1–3 minutes: focus on the pliability of your feet – pay particular attention to rolling through the foot and feeling the breadth of your foot, spreading as you roll.

3–5 minutes: become aware of your soft toes. Push off the big, middle and little toes evenly. You'll notice your pace increasing at this point.

6–9 minutes: keep your feet soft and mobile, but focus on how your ankles open up.

9–12 minutes: pull up and stabilise your hips – remember that tray of drinks.

12–15 minutes: concentrate on the relationship between your feet and hips – feel the muscles at the back of your legs beginning to work.

15–18 minutes: keep focusing on the feet and hips, but now layer in your long neck and your open, relaxed shoulders.

18–20 minutes: you are rolling through your feet with stable, lifted hips, long neck and relaxed shoulders – now think about those pendulum arms, swinging gently with each step.

20–25 minutes: keep walking. Focus on bringing the elbows back first, and getting the movement from the whole shoulder, rather than just the arm sockets. If it becomes a bit too difficult at this point, just focus on your pendulum arms again.

25–30 minutes: scan through your body as you keep each body part moving. Try to work out which parts of your body feel more comfortable and which feel stiff or awkward. (Make a mental note of this as we're going to build on it in Chapter Four: Just Do It.) Noticing what feels wrong is as important as noting what feels right.

Try not to get too hung up on timings – the minutes here are just a rough guide. The key is simply to layer in your body parts gradually. And if thirty to forty-five minutes feels too long, that's OK too – Give-it-a-go sessions can be as short as ten minutes (you just spend proportionately less time on each body part). But if you can manage longer, then do, as this will give you more time to really focus on putting it all together and feeling comfortable.

 TIP **Start from the bottom up**

If it feels like it's going wrong at any point (and it may well do), just come back to your feet. Start at the feet and build back up again, one body part at a time. Don't be tempted to work from the top down – if you do this, you will never get your alignment right. Always go from feet, to hips, to neck and shoulders, to arms. You may have to do this several times in the Give-it-a-go phase. That's normal. Just be patient and kind to yourself, and start back at your feet.

The point of Give-it-a-go is to appreciate the rhythm of a whole new, fluid way of walking. You aren't going to do this perfectly in these sessions, but you will begin to get glimmers of it all coming together – and at those moments, when your body works in harmony, you'll know how incredible Walkactive can be. Afterwards, you will feel that your whole body has exercised, rather than just your legs.

'The first time I felt it all come together well – and it was probably for about five seconds – I suddenly realised what all the fuss was all about! My movement, for those seconds, felt so natural and fluid and strong. I felt I was walking tall, but completely relaxed, using energy, without straining. It just felt right for my body – I wanted to walk that way for ever. Of course, a few moments later, I lost sight of what my feet were doing, and then I forgot to swing my arms and had to think about that again – it was mentally quite a challenge. But that glimpse – well, that was enough to show me that this was worth carrying on with – and I did. I now Walkactive with my dog for an hour every day and I've never felt fitter or stronger.'
LEE, 46, ATTENDED WALKACTIVE SPA BREAK

The Walkactive Dimmer Switch Effect

People often ask me if they're meant to do Walkactive all the time. The simple answer is YES! This is your new, youthful and effective way of walking. From now on, every step you take can and will be with the correct postural alignment. You might be thinking, 'Hang on a minute, there is no way I can walk like this all the time. What about when I am carrying bags or taking my children to school, walking slowly with elderly relatives, with colleagues at work or pushing a shopping trolley down the supermarket aisles?' The answer is you can! You just need to think in terms of a Walkactive dimmer switch.

Walkactive is not something you turn off and on ('Now I'm doing Walkactive, now I'm not'). Instead, you will become aware of Walkactive all the time. You may not be able to do the whole technique all the time, but you can always do aspects of it, such as the hip lift or symmetry of the torso. This means you are working on your body's amazing transformation all the time. We'll talk a lot more about different scenarios in later chapters, but for now you just need to gain the confidence and knowledge that will keep your Walkactive dimmer switch on at all times – simply turn it up or turn it down as and when you need to.

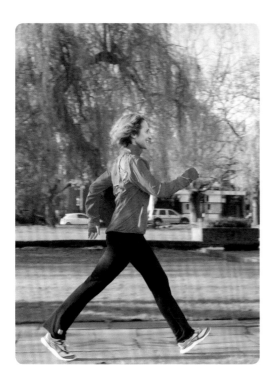

Pace

As you practise putting all the body parts together, your stride will get longer because you are pushing more through your toes. You may also notice a change in your pace. I talk about this in detail in Chapter Three, however pace is most definitely secondary to technique, so for now, don't worry about how fast or slow you're going – just focus on adding each body part in one by one and getting them all to work together smoothly. That said, try not to move too slowly, otherwise you'll never get into a rhythm and your movements will feel more stilted. Just see if you can find a pace that feels 'right' to you.

Don't forget your Technique Walks

You've done your two Give-it-a-go sessions, but I don't want you to forget about those shorter ten- to fifteen-minute Technique Walks (see page 30; your lunch break is a good place to start). In fact, I want you to keep practising on the individual body parts even when you know how to put all four together smoothly. Ongoing Technique Walks are a great way to remind yourself of what you are trying to do and how you need to do it. They are about getting it right. It's easy to forget parts of the technique or to get sloppy. Technique Walks are your insurance policy.

MAKING PROGRESS: HOW YOU MAY FEEL

How long it will take you to master the technique will depend on your fitness, mobility and body awareness. Having said that, it can help to have an idea of what you might expect to be feeling as you move through the first stages of learning Walkactive, so here is a rough guide:

After three days of Technique Walks

Session length: 10–15 minutes, three times per day

What you may feel: your feet feel a bit more natural when they're active – the foot is now more active than passive and strides are getting longer. In general, movements feel lighter, arms feel more natural.

After one week of Technique Walks

Session length: 10–15 minutes, three times per day

What you may feel: your body is moving in a more fluid way – when the session finishes you may not want to stop. You'll be starting to see benefits of Walkactive in other aspects of life too: you'll find you are standing better and maybe even sitting better at your desk or in the car.

 TIP ⋯⋯⋯⋯⋯⋯⋯⋯⋯⋯⋯⋯⋯⋯
Don't rush it

If you don't feel at all fluid, it's probably because you're rushing things. Don't just start walking and pick up your technique as if it's a basket of laundry – something you grab, and off you go. People often do this once they've understood the technique – they don't put the body parts together bit by bit any more. For best results, I want you to try to appreciate the mathematical sum of Walkactive – how adding each body part, one at a time, correctly, gives you the most amazing posture, joint alignment and shape change. This will bring fluidity.

After one Give-it-a-go session
Session length: 30–45 minutes

What you may feel: you'll probably feel a difference in the way you're moving, but your brain really has to concentrate. Your pace will improve, you'll feel more upright with less discomfort in the knees and hips and your calf muscles will start to contract, with some tightening of the muscles in your bottom.

 TIP *Go back to basics*

Mastering the swing of your arms may still feel a bit tricky, and adding them in might affect the other three parts of your technique. But your arms are the icing on the cake at this stage. So if you do find that adding them in throws off the other parts of your technique, stop! Lose the arms for now. Simply go back to focusing on your feet. Build up from the ground again: feet, hips, neck and shoulders. Then try adding in the arms. If it still doesn't work, go back to the feet again. Keep practising this. It may take time, but you'll get there with the arms if you think 'ground up' when it gets complicated.

YOU'RE OFF

You've now taken the first steps on your Walkactive journey – and you're off! Once you can put all the body parts together really well you can move on and focus on your particular goals, progressing as far as you like – even up to advanced levels of athletic training, if that's what you're after. But you will only get the results you long for, with no pain or stress, if you walk right!

And you'll have noticed that it isn't always easy – in fact, it can take a surprising amount of brain power and persistence. There is a Chinese expression that says, 'If you are experiencing frustration, then you are close to perfection!' You *will* master Walkactive, because thousands of other people just like you have done just that – they've toned up, grown longer, leaner, fitter, healthier and happier. They may even have added years to their lives, transforming not just their bodies, but the way they live.

So I want you to remember this, even when it feels complex or frustrating. What you are doing is not just another fad: this is intelligent exercise. Every single thing I'm asking you to do is rooted firmly in science and will improve any *body* of anyone of any age – from octogenarians to elite athletes. When your body walks the Walkactive way it changes. You change. So don't lose heart if it's not easy at first. Real change takes effort – but it's worth it!

CASE STUDY: KATHRYN – MASTERING THE TECHNIQUE, SEEING THE BENEFITS

Over the years Kathryn, aged fifty-two, had been serious about exercise. She'd gone to the gym regularly and done aerobics classes. She had always enjoyed walking, and known that it was good for her heath, but what she didn't realise was that walking 'right' could transform her body. Then she came on a one-day Walkactive course – she was hooked.

'With all my gym visits and aerobics, I had never experienced anything like the amazing body benefits I'm seeing now with Walkactive. At first my stride was quite quick and short. I was able to walk at what I thought was a good pace, but as soon as I started to put the Walkactive technique in place I felt the difference in my body.'

Kathryn found that she had to concentrate hard on working out her active feet – making her foot 'peel' off the ground rather than snatching it away. That took a few sessions to really get right. But once she'd mastered that, she began to see rapid results.

'The effort to master the technique is so worth it,' she says. 'Within four weeks I felt trimmer through my torso and felt I was walking a lot more smoothly. The technique has given me a lot more mobility in my hips and lower back, so I don't get the back discomfort I used to. Also, my husband says my bottom has definitely lifted and looks more pert – and as I am in my early fifties I'm very pleased about this!'

Kathryn joined her local Walkactive club, and is now a regular at Walk Time Trials. She loves the camaraderie and fun of Walkactive, but most of all she loves the results.

'I have never had as much body-shape change with any other form of exercise as I've had with Walkactive,' she says. 'And it's not just me; doing the courses with others you see the same changes happening all around you – with people of all different shapes, sizes, levels of motivation. It works for everyone, it really does.'

'The technique has given me a lot more mobility in my hips and lower back, so I don't get the back discomfort I used to.'

CHAPTER THREE

GETTING THE PACE RIGHT – FOR YOU

'...the most exciting thing was how natural and flowing the movement felt, even when I was walking really fast. I didn't want to stop – I just wanted to just keep on walking. I learned not to care how fast anyone else was going – it wasn't about that. It was about finding the right pace for me, and no one else. And what an amazing feeling!'

Pace is important. The right pace will help you achieve your specific health, weight-loss, cardiovascular or stamina goals. But don't panic – I'm not going to ask you to walk at a frantic sergeant-major speed with your arms punching wildly and stiffly through the air, nor am I going to ask you to walk at your fastest speed all the time. The really fabulous thing about Walkactive is that you don't have to achieve a 'set-in-stone' pace or push yourself beyond your capabilities. What you're going to do is find the pace that's *right for you* – the pace that will bring you the body transformation you long for, without strain or stress. And in so doing you'll gain not only speed but also confidence.

Best of all, however fast you go, you will still feel – and look – natural and relaxed. Think of a swimmer: as each of their hands enters the water it begins a stroke that will propel their body forward. And yet it looks effortless. The same goes for Walkactive: each time your foot touches down it begins the stride that will propel you over the ground. And, like a professional swimmer, you'll learn to propel your body faster, all the while maintaining a smooth, elegant and apparently effortless appearance. Even when your body is working hard, it will look effortless.

But it is not as simple as just saying to yourself, 'Right – I'm going to walk faster' or, 'I'm going to speed up'. You may well speed up, but when you do, your Walkactive technique could go out the window – and, if it does, your pace is irrelevant. So by far the most important thing to remember about pace is that it is always *secondary* to technique. If your technique isn't right, you can go as fast as you like, but you still won't get the full Walkactive body results. However, once you have mastered the Walkactive technique, you can train your

body to cover more distance with each stride. And when you find the right speed it's a bit like having one of those tried-and-tested recipes that you know always delivers – you follow it confidently, you enjoy the process and it brings amazing results.

PACE AND MUSCLES

As you may have gathered, I'm big on making your muscles work in a lengthened position. Mastering the correct Walkactive technique will teach your muscles to lengthen – and lengthened muscles generate more speed naturally, whatever

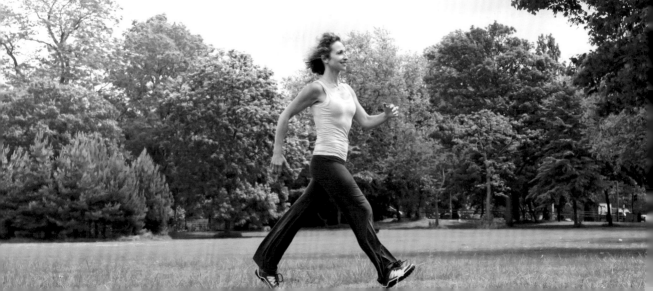

How Fast Do I Go?

People often ask me, 'How fast should I be walking?' There is actually no single answer to this question. Although your speed makes a difference to the number of calories you burn, to your strength, shape or cardiovascular fitness and to other goals you may have for your body, it's not just about moving at your fastest possible pace – fastest is not necessarily the best. Finding the pace that's right for you depends on what you want to get from Walkactive: do you want to be healthier overall, or to increase your cardiovascular stamina or to manage your weight? We'll explore these specific goals in more detail in the course of the next few chapters, but for now you need to focus on how to increase your pace without losing the technique.

your health, fitness or body shape. What's more, as you lengthen your muscles, your body also becomes more streamlined, and you move even faster.

There are a couple of analogies I use to explain exactly how and why this works. My clients find these really useful, and I think they'll help you too:

1. The Elastic Band Imagine you are holding a longish piece of elastic band between the thumb and first finger of your hand, so the band is neither stretched nor floppy. If you let one side of the elastic go the band doesn't snap back into place, it just flops. Now I want you to stretch that imaginary elastic band by moving your thumb and finger further apart, increasing the tension in the band. When you let go of one side, the band quickly snaps back to its original length – usually flying out of your hand. It has far more power because it has been stretched taut. The same goes for your muscles. What we are trying to do is lengthen them properly, before we ask them to contract and release. This way, when they spring back, they generate more power – and this power increases your pace.

2. The Bow and Arrow Imagine you have a bow and arrow in your hand. You're going to try to shoot at a target about 80 metres away. You draw your bow up and pull back the arrow, but you do not draw the arrow back as much as is possible, and you don't stretch the bow. You haven't created good tension before releasing the arrow. What will happen? Yes, the arrow's trajectory won't be straight, it will be more looped and limp and the arrow will flop down short of the target. Now imagine drawing that arrow back as far as possible until your bow is taut; aim at your target so that everything is aligned – the bow, the arrow – all in the right place, with the same intention, to hit that target. Now when you release the arrow it zooms off, much further, faster and with a straighter trajectory. This taut, aligned, lengthened ideal is what we are trying to achieve with Walkactive – and when you do, your body will travel further with each step you take. You'll walk faster!

'I have been practising the techniques more or less daily, and already I am aware that I am starting to tone up. Even more importantly, I am feeling less pressure on my knee and hip joints. At the moment I am still at the concentrating stage – and I really do have to concentrate – but I am determined to progress because I can see how beneficial this is for my whole body.'
ANJI, 60, ATTENDED WALKACTIVE ONE-DAY WORKSHOP

Fringe Benefits: Your Joint Health

What is doubly exciting about using your muscles properly to go faster is that when you do so you are no longer contracting and shortening the muscles around your joints, putting pressure on them. Instead, your joints have the space to move in the correct alignment. This means you don't just get a smoother, faster pace, you also protect your knee, hip and ankle joints. So the big extra payoff is that in addition to your body shape changing significantly because your pace is correct, your joints will be healthier and happier. It's win–win!

YOUR ACCELERATORS

So now that you appreciate the importance of lengthening your muscles, we need to look at your body's other natural 'internal accelerators' – the three parts of your body that are crucial when it comes to going faster. They are:

• your feet
• your hips
• your arms.

We've already looked at how these body parts should move correctly using my Walkactive technique. Now I'm going to teach you how to use all three of these as accelerators to increase your pace and further lengthen your muscles. You are going to work on making your feet even more pliable, so that they can propel you forward more powerfully. When your foot becomes more soft and pliable, and you really roll through it, pushing off your toes, you get more spring out of every step. This is what I call 'active' feet. You'll also keep your hips lifted, which allows your leg to extend further back with every step – and this uses the powerful muscles in your bottom more effectively. This longer stride will also allow you to cover more ground, faster. You'll learn to use your arms even more effectively too, so that they propel you forward as well.

Don't be intimidated by the idea of going faster

The work I'm asking you to do on accelerators applies to absolutely anyone, regardless of age, fitness, body shape or life stage. It can be tricky at first – some of the movements are quite subtle – but do persevere. This is about your body and your goals. I won't push you so that you injure or exhaust yourself. I am going to challenge your body – but safely, and intelligently. You'll feel yourself walking much faster, without stress or strain. It's a great feeling!

How to use your accelerators

To learn how to walk faster, you'll need to do some Technique Walks (see page 30), but this time focusing on using your three accelerators. I'm also going to ask you to do some drills to make sure you really understand the accelerator technique, and to establish the right pace for you.

As previously, focus on one body part per Technique Walk before you try to put your three accelerators together. It may take several ten- to fifteen-minute walks for you to really feel confident with one accelerator and appreciate how it speeds you up – but there is no rush. The better you are at the technique, the easier it will be to increase your pace. Indeed, as you master your accelerators, a faster pace will happen quite naturally!

Your feet

You already know that you are aiming to transform your foot from 'passive' to 'active'. Specifically, you are working to achieve an 'open ankle'. When it comes to pace, this open ankle is vital. So as you do your Technique Walks, try to:

- **push off your toes more** – remember, it's an even push, from the big, middle and little toes
- **keep your foot on the ground for longer** – the more contact there is between the surface of your foot and the ground, the more power you generate to propel yourself forward, and this is what makes you go faster
- **keep rolling through** *each part* **of your foot** (see below).

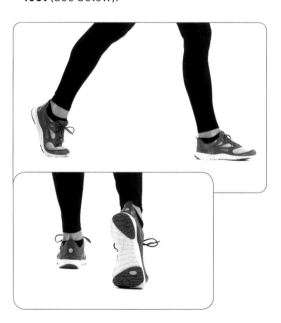

TIP ....

Watch out for tense feet

It is easy to tense the foot up when you are trying to move faster. But in fact, you want to do the opposite: you want to try and keep your foot relaxed and pliable (remember that plasticine – see page 31). The more pliable your foot is, the more pace you'll be able to generate out of each step.

Your hips

You are simply going to focus now on perfecting what you have already learned about the hips as this will automatically bring more power to your pace:

Hip stability without rigidity: a stable pelvis gives your muscles something to push against, and if they have something to push against, they can propel you faster across the ground. Imagine that swimmer again, pushing off the swimming-pool wall – if you have something stable to push against (in this case, your hips), you generate a stronger forward-moving power.

Hip lift: if your hips are lifted, then your hip joint can move more freely. This allows your thigh to extend further behind you with each stride. This backward extension of your thigh allows the big muscles in your bottom to contract more fully, propelling you forward more powerfully. The result is a faster speed (and a toned bottom!).

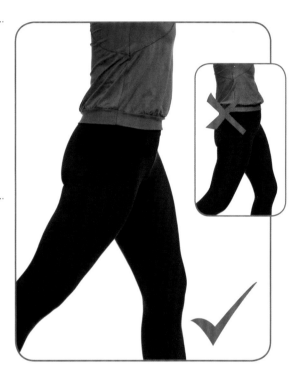

The Science: Why Hip Stability Makes You Go Faster

When your hips are stable, the big power-generating muscles in your bottom (your glutes) can contract – or push – against them. As you push off your toes, keeping your hips stable, your muscles push against your pelvis, propelling you forward faster. If, on the other hand, your hips and midriff are slack and loose, these important big muscles have nothing to contract against. You therefore lose power, pace and, ultimately, tone.

It's little wonder that I like to pay so much attention to this hip area; it affects how you look, move, the number of calories you burn – and how fast you go.

TROUBLESHOOTING

'My hips and thighs feel tight now!' When you start to master your feet and hip accelerators you may well feel that the front part of your hips and the front of your thighs get a bit stiff or sore. This is because your hips are actually starting to work! They are – at last – achieving their correct, full range of motion. This, in turn, is asking those big muscles down the front of your legs (your quadriceps) to stretch more too. But they are still tight and too short. It'll take time to lengthen and stretch them.

So stick with it because as your range of motion improves your stride will lengthen, allowing you to cover more ground and faster. And, as an added bonus, what you are doing will help to reduce back discomfort and improve your posture. In short, a bit of discomfort in the hips or front of your thighs at this stage is a great sign!

Your arms

You already know that as your arms swing, you need to focus more on the backward movement, letting them swing naturally forward again. To help you walk faster, try to make sure that you really focus on making your arms swing from the shoulder muscles that run across your upper back (the shoulder girdle), rather than just moving from the shoulder joint at the top of your arm. There is a circular effect here: the shoulder movement allows your torso to gently rotate as you walk, and this rotation helps you to move faster. The faster you walk, the more your arms will swing, and this swing will also propel you forward.

Stride length

You may have noticed that so far I have not talked about how long your stride should be. This is deliberate. As you begin to walk faster, using your natural accelerators, your strides will probably lengthen of their own accord. This will be as a natural *consequence* of using your feet, hips and arms to generate speed,

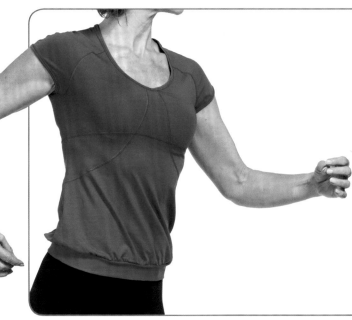

rather than because you are trying to force yourself to go faster. If you try to force your stride to lengthen, then you are likely to use all the wrong muscles again – those at the front of your legs, to pull you forward, rather than those in your bottom and down the back of your legs – to propel you.

This is why I have kept quiet about stride length. I want you to enjoy how your stride changes naturally, rather than forcing it. If you do this, you'll start to move faster while still looking natural – as if you are gliding along, smoothly and effortlessly across the ground.

CASE STUDY: KATE – GETTING ACTIVE

In January 2011 Kate had had enough. She was overweight, tired and run down. Just a short walk to the shops left her short of breath, and her doctor had advised her to get back in shape or she'd face serious health issues.

With the New Year had come the usual resolution to lose weight and get fit. But this time, she didn't try a new diet or buy a gym membership that would never be used. Instead, she signed up for Walkactive.

Just five months later, Kate had lost 7 stone (44.5kg). And two years on, she's kept that weight off. She can now walk up five flights of stairs at work with hardly a puff. She feels fit, toned and healthy and recently walked 7 kilometres in a remarkable forty-eight minutes.

'Right from the start, I felt really encouraged,' says Kate. 'It took a while for the technique to sink in, but once it did, it just felt like a really natural way to move. You can get into a rhythm which is really stress-busting. My whole body shape has changed now. I feel incredibly toned and, best of all, I have rediscovered my waist! I am still constantly surprised by how much I can do now – for instance, I recently went on a bike ride for the first time in years and it felt fantastic. Walkactive has been the most positive thing I have done in a long time. And it's so much nicer going around the park seeing all the seasons, than being stuck in a gym.'

PICK UP YOUR PACE: THREE PACE DRILLS TO TRY NOW

I'm going to take you through a combination of standing and moving drills that will help you to use the techniques I've explained and improve your Walkactive pace. These drills are not designed to be performed at full speed. Think of them as an addition to your Technique Walks – something you practise regularly. They are simply extra ways to help you improve your technique and, therefore, your pace. If you do your drills, you'll see results quicker!

Drill 1: open ankle

Aim: to help you appreciate the difference between an open ankle and a closed one, so you know what to aim for. It also helps you to notice how you are lengthening through your leg muscles in order to improve your pace.

How to do it
- Stand with good posture, shoulders back and down, neck long, feet hip-width apart.
- Take a large step back with your right foot – as if you are doing a calf stretch. You should be able to feel a slight stretch on your right calf – if you don't, then try to take that leg slightly further back.

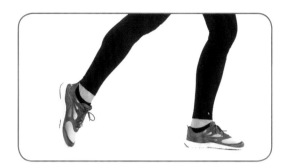

- From here, bring your weight more on to your front (left) foot. Now roll through your back (right) foot, so that you are leaning on the tips of those toes – as if you're on a ballet point. You should feel unstable in this position, as your balance is going to be challenged. Try to notice how your right leg is long and extended and your hip is open at the front. This is *not* an open-ankle position.

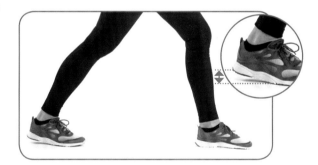

- Next, lower the right foot, but keep the heel off the floor (see above): your toes, the ball of your right foot and the arch should be in contact with the floor, but not your heel. Notice how your ankle is 'closed' – it is at more of a right angle to your foot. This is *not* an open ankle either.

- Now ease forward from this position until you are rolling on to the ball of your foot, just before your toes begin – as if you are standing on your highest tiptoe. This *is* your open ankle. In this position (see below), you should feel stable. Your right leg should be long. Your hip and pelvis area should feel open and you should also feel balanced. You should have an awareness of your big, middle and little toes.
- Repeat this drill on the other foot.

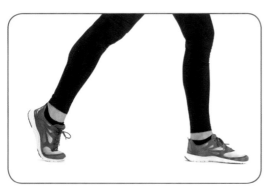

TIP **Keep checking your position**

You may feel as if you are coming all the way forward into an open ankle as you walk, but if you have been sitting at a desk all day or driving a car, then the chances are your ankles will be stiff – their range of motion will be limited, even if you've been practising your Technique Walks. So after you've been walking for about ten minutes, try to do a few more open-ankle drills. This will help you to check your position and technique.

Drill 2: hip lift

Aim: to help you get into a correct hip-lift position. Correctly lifted hips will lengthen the muscles in your bottom (the glutes), and – as you know all too well from your elastic band or your bow and arrow (see page 51) – a lengthened muscle will generate more power each time you push off your toes. A good hip lift also allows your hip extensor muscles to extend fully – this lets you take a longer stride with each step, rather than taking lots of little short steps.

How to do it

- Move into your open-ankle position, as above. From there, lengthen your upper torso in and up, pulling away from your hips, as if you are doing those Abdominal J exercises (on page 37). The idea here is to lift up and out of your hips, rather than to sit into your pelvis and hips like a sack of potatoes. If it helps, place your fingers on your hips and ribcage and feel the space between the two (see opposite). You are trying to apply my bow-and-arrow concept – pre-lengthening your muscles to achieve propulsion, that springing-forward movement.
- Now pay attention to your shoulders – check that they do not rise. Also, check that your ribcage has not expanded. To do this, try to focus on drawing in and up from the hips, but at the same time

allow your shoulders to be soft and your neck to be long. If it helps, imagine I am with you, resting my hands gently on your shoulders: you want to make sure those dangly earrings have space to be seen (see page 39).

- Hold this position for a count of twenty: you should feel taller and you may well feel more of a stretch and opening down the front of your hips. Your abdominals will also feel more taut and your front thigh muscles will feel taut and lengthened.
- Repeat twice on each side.

'At first I really found it hard to understand the idea of pulling my hips up – on the day of the workshop I still hadn't cracked it. But I kept going and I noticed that it became much easier the more I used the foot part of the technique. What you realise is that it's all connected – this really is intelligent exercise. Amazingly, I've also noticed that my posture is now much better when sitting as well as walking.'
PAM, 56, ATTENDED WALKACTIVE ONE-DAY WORKSHOP

Drill 3: arm swing

Aim: to help you appreciate how your arms can propel you forward. Note: you do this drill standing still!

How to do it

- Stand with a good posture. Apply your Abdominal J (see page 37) so that you feel yourself lifting up and out of your hips (as above). Remember to relax your shoulders, giving those dangly earrings or rulers plenty of space.
- Now add a small bend at the elbow. Start to swing your arms backward and forward, paying attention to the back swing – it should be larger than the front swing – and remembering to lead with your elbow on the back swing (not your hand).
- Start to speed up the arm swing, still concentrating on swinging more backward

than forward. As you do so you'll probably want to move forward – this is simple physics: the more power you generate on the back swing the more the body will want to propel itself forward.

When I'm working with clients I will often ask them to try and swing the elbow back far enough to touch my hand, as below. It may help to envisage a hand behind you that you are trying to touch.

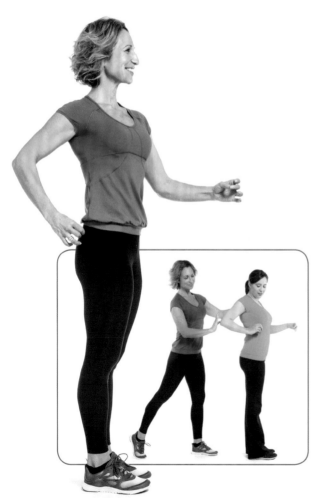

Drill 4: the whole-body accelerator

Aim: to help you appreciate how each of your body's natural accelerators contributes to your pace. It also helps you to put your accelerators together.

How to do it

- Find a flat, level area with some kind of markers – these can be an avenue of trees or benches or lampposts positioned about twelve to thirty paces apart, or you can use cones or any other recognisable marker. Don't place them any further than thirty paces apart though – any more than this and you may find that your attention drifts. You're going to focus on a different accelerator at each new marker so you need to be able to really concentrate on each one.

- Now start walking. Begin by concentrating on using your feet to get more pace into your Walkactive technique: gently push off your toes and absorb the ground with your whole foot at each stride. Keep your attention on building your pace through your feet until you come level with the next marker. This is your cue to add in the next natural body accelerator – your hips.

- You are still going to use your feet, but now you add in your hip lift. Try to gain more pace without compromising your Walkactive technique (so keep the arms

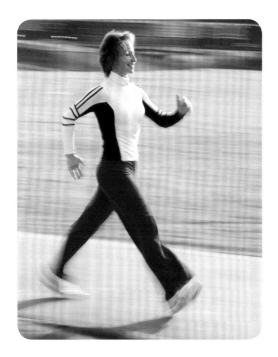

out of it for the moment). Feel how your stride lengthens and the muscles in your bottom contract. Keep this going until you reach the third marker.

- Now you're going to add your third natural body accelerator – your arms. Let your arms swing naturally. Focus on the back swing, and on keeping the swing coming all the way into the shoulder girdle. Speeding up your arm swing will naturally help your legs to move faster without shortening your stride.
- Repeat this drill twice. As you put it all together, you should feel that your body is starting to move more naturally. You'll notice that you're going faster without your technique looking snatched or stiff.

- Try to relax. Check that your feet are not tense. Your movement should be fluid and flowing. Well done – you are now doing it! This is Walkactive with pace. Next we'll need to decide exactly how fast you should go.

TROUBLESHOOTING

'It feels jarring!' If, as you try to speed up, you feel tense or strained and your strides get shorter this is a sure sign that you are using the wrong muscles and at the wrong time (you'll feel as if all the muscles in your legs and bottom are contracting all the time, rather than a muscle contracting and then relaxing again). If this happens – and it often does when you are getting used to walking faster – then stop. Go back to your Walkactive basic technique – start at the feet and revisit each of the four body parts in turn. Try to appreciate how each part impacts on the next. Then, when you have this, move on to your accelerators, feeling how each part of the accelerators works – feet, hips, arms.

'I was amazed that when I managed to put all my accelerators together – and believe me, it took some practice – I started to walk so much faster without actually thinking about it. I was concentrating on the elements of the technique, but before I knew it, I was covering much more ground – and it felt amazing.'
JOY, 45, ATTENDED WALKACTIVE SPA BREAK

FIND YOUR OPTIMUM WALKING PACE (OWP)

This is a crucial part of Walkactive. It will determine the speed you walk at, and it will make a huge difference to the results you see.

Your Optimum Walking Pace (OWP) is the fastest you can walk without compromising your technique. There might be a temptation to walk really fast, but always remember: technique is what matters most. If you are walking so fast that you just can't keep your technique going then you won't revolutionise your body. You'll just get tired and fed up (and worse, you might do yourself some actual damage).

Everyone has their own OWP. Yours should be achievable and sustainable – but also challenging (and again, not at the expense of your technique). In order to find your OWP, you need to do the following break-point drill.

Break-point drill

For this drill you need a long stretch of space where you can walk without interruption. Make sure you have thoroughly warmed up first – go through all the four parts of your basic Walkactive technique for at least ten minutes. You also need about six to eight markers. Again, it's fine to use lampposts, benches or evenly spaced trees.

- Start walking from the first to the second marker at a leisurely pace, but with a good Walkactive technique. When you are level with your second marker, increase your pace, using your body accelerators – feet, hips, arms (see pages 53–5).
- Keep this constant increased pace until you reach the third maker. When you get there, increase your pace again.
- Continue increasing your pace at each marker until you feel you are walking so fast that you have to break into a jog. This is your break point. Every one of us has a different break point. It is partly influenced by fitness, partly by technique and partly by ability.
- The pace you were walking at just before you reached your break point is your Maximum Walking Pace. This isn't the same as your OWP! At your Maximum Walking Pace, your technique will have gone to pieces. All your lovely correct postural alignment will have disappeared and you'll be flailing. But don't worry. It is important to recognise how uncomfortable and 'wrong' this feels – this is an important part of identifying the OWP.
- So to find your OWP, repeat the break-point drill, but this time, once you hit your break point, ease off your Maximum Walking Pace by about 5 to 10 per cent – just enough that you can reclaim your Walkactive technique. *This* is your OWP.

'I've been doing Walkactive for a year now, and I'm in better shape than I've been in years, but I do find that I have to remind myself, frequently, of my OWP. I still do the break-point drill quite often, and it stops me getting complacent. I think this has been one of the greatest keys to success: my drills. They keep me focused and stop me slacking off!'

SALLY, 62, JOINED A LOCAL WALKACTIVE GROUP

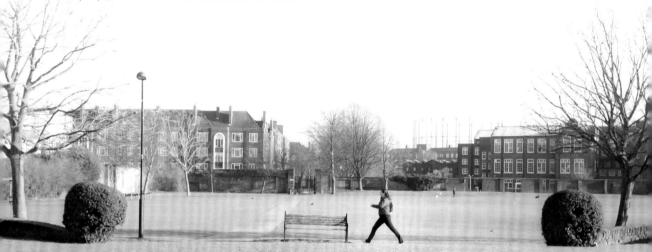

TIP ***Do the drills more than once***

I suggest that you repeat the break-point drill several times to find your OWP. I guarantee that the first time you do it the break point you find will not be your true break point! You'll need to give it a few goes. The more you do it, the more likely that you will be able to find the real point – that definitive speed at which you are out of control. Finding this point will give you something concrete to work on.

Remember – this is about *you*

Your OWP should be fast enough that you are breathless, but slow enough that you can maintain a good technique. When you are starting out, repeat the break-point drill at the beginning of every walk. This will get you used to how your OWP really feels. Your OWP will increase as you get fitter – so don't compare it with anyone else's or worry that it's too slow. Remember, this is about what Walkactive can do for you. So explore how fast you can go, without losing your vital technique.

AM I WALKING FAST ENOUGH?

To answer this question you need to identify your OWP – and keep going. Here's how: once you have done the break-point drill several times, repeat it once more. But this time don't stop. Carry on walking for about ten or fifteen minutes using your three natural accelerators. Try to ensure the pace is smooth but effective, challenging but sustainable. You should feel out of breath, but not completely breathless – you should be able to carry on a conversation, but not too easily. Aim for a consistent pace, rather than bursts or fits and starts. This will take a few attempts. You may indeed find that your pace fluctuates at first, but don't panic. I'm going to help you to build on this in the next few chapters! And remember, if you do find that your pace feels difficult or painful or stressful, always go back to your technique. Start with the feet and move up, body part by body part. Get it right. That's by far the most important thing.

PACE WALKS – TIME TO GET MOVING!

Pace Walks are similar in principle to Technique Walks. But now your focus is on getting more of a cardiovascular effect: you're going to improve the stamina of your heart and lungs by walking faster for longer.

To start with, allocate fifteen to twenty minutes in which to work on your pace:

• For the first five to ten minutes, focus on your three accelerators – as you did on pages 53–5 – this time putting them together.
• When you've done this, stop, and do a couple of break-point drills.
• Now, focusing on your three accelerators again, start to walk at your OWP. See if you can do this for just ten minutes at first. For now you're just building up your ability to walk at a faster pace, and getting used to how that faster pace feels.
• Try to do three or four of these Pace Walks over the course of the week – where you simply get used to walking at a good strong pace for longer.

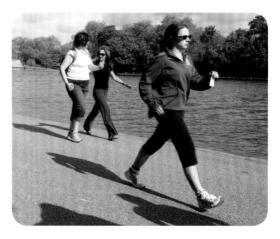

MOVING FORWARD

In the next few chapters you'll learn about adjusting your pace and the duration of your walks in order to achieve your specific goal, whether it's inch loss, better health or increased fitness. I'll also teach you how you can use your different speeds depending on the situation you're in, and what you are trying to achieve. For now, to help you visualise how different Walkactive paces can work for you, here is a brief overview:

Posture pace

What is it? You are applying your Walkactive basic technique, but your accelerators are not switched on. You get toning, joint health and postural benefits from this pace.

When to use it: this is how you'll mostly move around during the day – at home, at work, perhaps on your walk to work or along the supermarket shopping aisles. Your Walkactive technique is in place, but your accelerators are not on. In other words, the Walkactive switch is on but the dimmer (see page 45) is turned to low.

Technique pace

What is it? You are applying your basic Walkactive technique and your accelerators are switched on – this is faster than posture pace and working towards OWP, though exactly how fast you are going will depend on which part of the technique you are working on.

When to use it: during your drills and Technique Walks.

Optimum Walking Pace (OWP)

What is it? This is your cardiovascular-training and fitness-training pace: you're using your basic techniques and your accelerators to walk as fast as you can, without compromising technique.

When to use it: on your Pace Walks – when you are teaching yourself to walk faster for longer.

Maximum Walking Pace

What is it? This, as its name suggests, is the fastest possible pace you can walk at. Your technique will have gone completely out the window and you'll be using all the wrong muscles in the wrong way – and at the wrong time. You'll feel tense, rigid and stiff and slightly out of control. This is not Walkactive – it's more like power walking.

When to use it: never! Or at least only *ever* use this pace when doing your break-point drill.

'I've never been a fast walker by any means, but I found that my pace had increased significantly even by day two of my two-day residential programme. I was really amazed by what I was capable of. It did take me a while to find my Optimum Walking Pace, but when I got used to that speed by doing my Pace Walks, the most exciting thing was how natural and flowing the movement felt, even when I was walking really fast. I didn't want to stop – I just wanted to just keep on walking. I learned not to care how fast anyone else was going – it wasn't about that. It was about finding the right pace for me, and no one else. And what an amazing feeling! When it's right, I feel as if my body is gliding along. It's hard work, definitely. I'm out of breath and I get very warm, so I'm not coasting, but it doesn't feel stressful or awkward at all.'

GEETHA, 56, ATTENDED A WALKACTIVE TWO-DAY RESIDENTIAL COURSE

Geetha has learned what so many people learn with Walkactive – that picking up the pace is not a painful, stressful experience. It stretches you and you have to work at it, but it feels really good. And it looks effortless. As your pace increases – and it will naturally, as you perfect the technique and work on your accelerators – you'll enjoy more and more fluidity too. You really will glide.

But as I always tell people, Walkactive isn't just about what feels right, it's also about learning *what feels wrong*. As you work on speeding up, you will get to know your body. You'll connect with it on a much deeper level than you have before, and you'll start to listen to how it feels. The more you understand your body and tune into it, the faster this learning process will be.

It's all too easy for your Walkactive technique to slip as you speed up. This happens to everyone at first. But if you're tuned into how your body feels when you walk right, then you'll be able to correct yourself when your technique slips. When you walk 'wrong' it will, quite simply *feel* wrong.

Conversely, when Walkactive is right, it's really right: you will use your accelerators to speed up, lengthen your strides and muscles and really use your body with effort, but without strain. This really is an amazing feeling and once you've got it, you can achieve anything you want for your body!

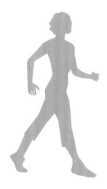

CHAPTER FOUR

JUST DO IT

'My shape has changed dramatically – I've lost over a stone [6.4kg] and 4 inches [10cm] off my waist – but it has never felt like a struggle. The amazing thing for me is that I don't want to stop. There's no willpower involved; this is just who I am now.'

By now, you should have had glimmers of how amazing Walkactive can feel. You are changing the habits of a lifetime and, as you progress, these glimmers will increase. Soon you'll find the benefits of Walkactive transferring themselves to other aspects of your life. Without even thinking about it, you will begin to move correctly as you potter around the house or the office, or even as you sit at your computer. Your muscles will lengthen and tone with every step you take throughout your day, even when you're not specifically doing a Walkactive session. This is called the 'embedding phase', where Walkactive is becoming subconscious. Your internal framework is changing to become taut, long and lean, and your baggy muscles are vacuum-packing themselves around this framework. This is why Walkactive is different from an 'exercise routine' – you're learning to move 'right' without even thinking about it, and then you'll move this way for life.

But getting to this stage is not always plain sailing. In fact, Walkactive – like any change of habit – can take determination, planning and confidence. There will be times

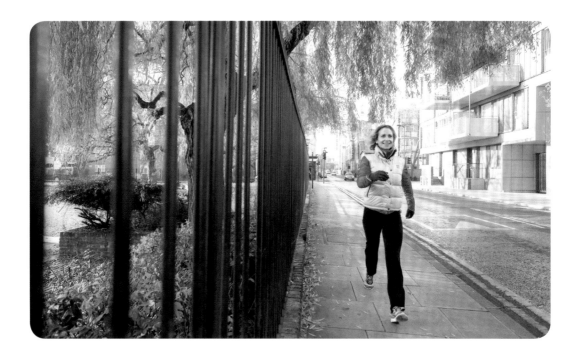

when it seems too much, and times when you aren't sure it's working out.

If you feel daunted by this, don't panic because that's exactly what we are going to look at in this chapter: we are going, as Nike say, to *just do it* – and then we're going to *just keep doing it*.

THE RIGHT TIME TO START

Just doing it *at all* is your first major hurdle. You may want to wait until you have a clear stretch in your diary where life looks simpler and you can really give Walkactive your full attention. But you know what? That time is never going to come. The perfect time to just do it is *now* – whatever else is going on in your life. The first step is to transform your mindset from 'I'm going to do this' into 'I'm doing this – right now'.

Set yourself up for success ...

Walkactive is about your body, for sure, but it's also about your mind. It's about building confidence, believing that you can do this and that it's working for you – that it's becoming a part of who you are. One of the biggest hurdles is going to be your expectations. You may have decided that you're going to push Walkactive to the absolute max, every single day, whatever is happening, so you can transform yourself as quickly as possible. I totally love the idea you are going to immerse yourself in Walkactive. Go for it – it is *so* worth it! But at the same time, I do want you to be realistic about what you can achieve, week by week, in the *real world*. And to do this, you have to be honest, look ahead and plan.

So at the start of each week I want you to sit down and look at the week ahead. What do the next seven days have in store for you? How much Walkactive will you be able to do, realistically? Is this one of those weeks when life is going to get fraught? Maybe you're moving house or have a huge report to submit at work, or it's the children's half term, or your mother isn't very well. These are all valid reasons why it's going to be hard to fit Walkactive sessions into your week. And if you ignore this reality, you are likely to end up feeling like a failure.

However, it's not a case of just *not* doing it. Oh no – what you're going to do is shape your expectations about what's achievable for you this week. So even if it's just five minutes per day as you walk to the bus stop, or making sure your technique is right as you move around the house, you must do something. Maybe you walk a considerable part of your journey to work already. You may not need to find masses of 'spare' time – but you can optimise the time you have already. Walkactive is *always* possible.

A clear picture of what's achievable for you will help to build your confidence that you really can do this. You'll realise that it's possible to fit Walkactive into your life whatever is happening. It's a bit like that dimmer switch: you don't switch Walkactive on and off according to how busy you are, but you might have to turn the intensity down.

So now look at the coming week and try to classify it as one of the following:

- **A progressive week** If it looks as though you'll have lots of time for Walkactive – you're confident that you can achieve all the Technique Walks, drills and Pace Walks that you'd like to do – then it's a progressive week. It's a week when your Walkactive will improve, you'll feel changes, you'll feel like you're getting somewhere. In a progressive week, you are 85 to 95 per cent confident you can achieve your Walkactive goals.
- **A maintenance week** The week ahead is busy: you've got relatives staying, or a big work commitment, or a busy social schedule. You think you'll be able to do some Walkactive, but not as much as you'd like. This then is a maintenance week. You're going to do enough to maintain your efforts – you'll keep up your technique, maybe even take a Pace Walk

or two. You'd like to do more, but this is valuable too – you're being consistent, you're turning Walkactive into a reality and you're cementing your technique.

- **A damage-limitation week** The coming week looks overwhelming: you're moving house, you've got the builders in, a relative is ill. This is a damage-limitation situation. Instead of throwing in the towel and waiting for life to calm down, you're going to limit the damage and do a little bit. This isn't anywhere near what you'd want to do, but it's something. Doing *something* will stop you from feeling you can't possibly manage Walkactive. It will make you realise that Walkactive is possible. And gradually, you'll find that even in damage-limitation weeks, you'll find ways to do much more than you'd hoped.

...then review your week

Once you've got through the week, look back on it, before you plan out the next week. You'll be surprised at how things turn out. What you might have felt would be a damage-limitation week could have turned out to be a maintenance week. Or perhaps you planned a progressive week, but unexpected things happened – the washing machine flooded, you were clobbered by a new deadline at work or other unexpected demands landed on your plate – and it became a damage-limitation week. If this happens – and it almost certainly will sometimes – you can simply draw a line under it. Be aware that rather than giving Walkactive up, you've found ways to fit it into your life even in small chunks. And the more your confidence builds about your ability to do this, the more easily you'll find ways to do it.

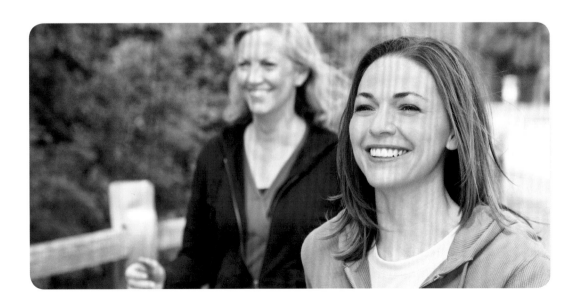

YOUR MINDSET: SUCCESS VERSUS FAILURE

You will see and feel the benefits of Walkactive across all aspects of your life, even when you're sitting at a computer or behind the wheel of a car. That's what makes my technique so unique and effective. But to do this you have to change the way you think about exercise. Some of the effort involved in Walkactive is going to be mental, not physical.

Your Template of Failure

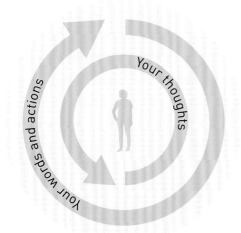

The chances are that you've started exercise plans in the past and dropped them because they just weren't sustainable. You want the quick fix, and at first you're prepared to suffer for it. You say, 'I'm going to do this', and you do it. Initially it works, but in the back of your mind you are thinking: 'I'm never going to keep this up. I'm going to end up back where I started.' What you *say* and *do* are moving in one direction. But what you *think* is going in completely the opposite direction. Soon, you give up. You think, 'Here we go again', and before long any results have reversed themselves and you're back at square one, looking for the next quick fix.

This pattern of success/failure, where your thoughts work against you, erodes your confidence and your self-esteem. And if you do it a few times, you start to believe you'll never achieve your goal. This is your 'Template of Failure'.

Your Template of Success

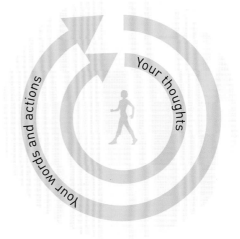

What you need to do, right now, is erase that Template of Failure once and for all and nurture a Template of Success instead.

When life gets busy you may indeed stop *doing* some parts of Walkactive. You may even stop *saying* that you're changing your life. But your *thoughts* are always in the right place – they remain positive, building and nurturing your confidence. You're still *thinking* 'I can do this' – even on days when the plan is hard to maintain. Walkactive is a powerful way to nurture this Template of Success because it doesn't impose a strict and unsustainable routine. Walkactive puts *you* in control:

- *You* decide what you want to achieve – for example, good health, fitness, inch loss or weight management.
- *You* assess whether your life right now allows your plan for the week to be a progressive, maintenance or damage-limitation one.
- *You* select the approach that best fits your needs and life *right now.*
- *You* appreciate that you can do more, or less, but that the Walkactive dimmer switch is always on.

'I set out with great intentions, I was going to walk 7500 steps per day, and do all my Pace Walks and lose 5 inches [12.5cm]. For the first two weeks I was totally determined and focused, and I made it work – I found ingenious ways to increase my steps, and I made myself do the Pace Walks even when I was tired. But then, in week three, I had to travel unexpectedly for work, I had several crazy deadlines and then my youngest child, aged five, was at home sick for two days. I couldn't plan for any of this. What I thought was going to be a progressive week turned into a wipeout. In the past, if this sort of thing had happened with an exercise regime, I'd have thought, "Right that's it, this just isn't going to work, I can't do this." And I'd have given up. But because I knew about progressive/maintenance and damage-limitation weeks I just did what I could. I made it out for one ten-minute Pace Walk, and though my steps were nowhere near 7500 per day, I did manage to find ways to up them a bit – walking around while on the phone, walking round the house, up and down stairs, doing my Abdominal Js. I limited the damage. But most of all, I realised it was OK – it was a bad week, but I didn't need to give up. Since then, I've kept it up. There've been good weeks and bad weeks, but I've lost my 5 inches, gone down to a size ten from a size fourteen and I feel radically better. People tell me I look ten years younger! My life hasn't changed – it's as bonkers as ever – but my mindset definitely has.'

SUSIE, 45, ATTENDED WALKACTIVE SPA BREAK

WHAT YOU NEED TO 'JUST DO IT'

I'll talk about your general kit – clothing, shoes, bags – later in this chapter, but for now, the number-one piece of Walkactive kit that you need is a pedometer.

A pedometer is essential to your Walkactive success – it is going to become your best friend.

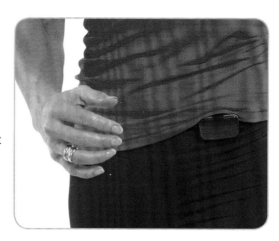

What is a pedometer – and why do I need one?

A pedometer is a device about the size of a matchbox that typically attaches to your belt or waistband and counts your walking or running steps. It is going to help you reach your target, track your progress and keep on going.

Which one should I buy?

Some pedometers can be kept in a shirt pocket or a bag. Some can calculate and display other interesting statistics such as distance, calories burned, speed, elapsed time, steps per minute. Some will function as a stopwatch and an alarm, others have fancy features such as talking, playing music or reading your heart rate. With developing technology pedometers are changing fast – you can buy shoes or wrist bands where they are built in or you can get technology for your Smartphone (an 'app').

But yours doesn't have to be fancy. When it comes to choosing a pedometer there are two things that really matter: it should accurately record how many steps you take, and it should calculate your step rate (i.e. how many steps you take per minute). Historically, pedometers are most accurate when it comes to counting steps, less so at calculating distance walked, and even less at estimating how many calories you have burned. This is fine though, since the latest scientific research shows that the number of steps you take is more important than the distance you travel. And with Walkactive you'll burn plenty of calories – so don't worry about that!

Pedometers as motivators

In a 2005 study in Knoxville, Tennessee, a group of women were given pedometers. Half of them could see their pedometers and were told to aim for 10,000 steps per day. The other group couldn't see theirs, and were told to aim for sixty to eighty minutes' brisk walking per day. The women in the group who could read their pedometer at any time managed 10,000 steps per day more often than the others who took, on average, only about 8000 steps per day – that's a difference of 1 mile (1.6km) every day. Even on days when they didn't make their targets, the group who could see their pedometers walked more than those who couldn't. Pedometers, in other words, have hidden motivational benefits.

How Do I Know If My Pedometer is Accurate?

You'd be surprised at how inaccurate pedometers can be. Some are worse than useless! One way to test a pedometer's accuracy is to perform a twenty-step test. To do this, attach your pedometer to your belt or waistband in line with your knee (it doesn't matter which side). Reset it to zero. Take twenty steps at your typical walking pace. Check to see if the pedometer reads between eighteen and twenty-two steps. If it does, that means it is likely to be a reasonably accurate step counter. (Bear in mind that in general, most pedometers are fairly accurate step counters at speeds of 2.5mph and above. Even some of the most accurate pedometers miscount steps at slower speeds.) If not, reposition it on your belt or waistband, and do the test again. If it repeatedly fails this test, it is not accurate.

 TIP ···· *Ensuring your pedometer's accuracy*

Studies have shown that a variety of factors can affect a pedometer's step-counting accuracy. Pedometers are generally more accurate if you attach them to a firm waistband in an upright position. They tend to underestimate steps if you attach them to a loose waistband. Your pedometer may also be less accurate if it is tilted or at an angle – in fact, studies show that if you have a large belly, and the pedometer therefore sits at an angle, this can affect its accuracy. If this applies to you, try moving your pedometer to the side or even to the back of your trousers, then double-checking its accuracy. Alternatively, you could even try clipping it to your sock.

ESTABLISH YOUR STARTING POINT

To make Walkactive work for you, in your life – real life – it's important to establish where you're starting from. So I want you to take a good look at your life and your activity levels.

Ask yourself: how active am I – *right now*? You may think, 'I'm a pretty active person'. But are you – really? Have a think about this: it is 7pm and you are finally flopping down. You feel tired, it's been a busy day, and you've been 'active'. But what was the activity? Was it:

- **physical**: you've walked a long way, played lots of sport, moved boxes all day or spent the whole day digging in the garden – you have moved your body a lot
- **mental**: your brain has been madly busy – you've had reports at work to write, you've had to organise a family event, cover for an absent colleague, cope with a mini crisis at home or run the house (involving feeding a family, supervising homework or squabbles, doing the online weekly shop, calling the plumber); you've been 'on the go' the whole time, but has your body moved much?
- **travel-based**: you have been across town after dropping the children at school, picked up the dry cleaning, rushed to the office for a meeting, collected your weekly food shop, fetched the parcel from the post office, presented at your company's board meeting, then rushed back to see your son play in his afternoon sports fixture. You've covered a lot of ground, but mainly by car, train, bus, taxi, escalator – in fact, in all sorts of ways that have not really involved moving your body. The truth is, while you're tired and you've covered a long distance, you've barely taken a step!

The bottom line here is that the only way to know how much you've moved is to record your actual number of steps. You'll be amazed at the difference between how active you feel and how active you actually are. So to establish where you are now you need to work out how many steps you take during an average day (your 'average daily baseline') and how many steps you take per minute (your 'step rate').

How to find your average daily baseline

To do this you need to wear an accurate pedometer for three consecutive days and walk the way you always walked before you knew a thing about Walkactive. Again, don't wait for three clear days when you know you'll walk a lot. This is real life – your life – and we're talking about your body, right now, not some idealised version of yourself.

So start now
- At the start of each day put on your pedometer. Check that it's set at zero.
- Wear the pedometer all day until you go to bed. At the end of the day, write down how many steps you have done in the chart on page 76 or write it down in a notebook. Repeat this on the following two days, so you have three daily readings.
- Add the three readings together and divide by three to find your average number of daily steps. This is your baseline.

How to find your step rate

Go to a stretch of smooth pathway that will allow you to walk uninterrupted for sixty seconds.

- Set your pedometer to zero and start walking normally (the pace at which you usually walked around in your daily life before you started learning the Walkactive technique – for instance, the way you'd walk from your bedroom to the bathroom, or down the supermarket aisle). Walk 'normally' for sixty seconds and then stop.
- Check your pedometer and make a note of your step rate.

 TIP *Keep it real*

Make sure you really do walk as you normally would (i.e. your pre-Walkactive style) – don't speed up and don't try to use the Walkactive technique. You need to establish a true picture of how you actually walk right now – not a picture of how well you can walk, or how far. This honest information will be your solid starting point. If you are realistic, you'll be able to see clearly where you need to go to achieve your goals and you'll be able to monitor your progress. The more accurate you are with this information, the more successful you will be with Walkactive.

Keeping a record

Use the charts below to record where you are at right now – how many steps on average you take each day and at what rate. Alternatively, you can jot them down in a notebook.

My daily baseline record

	Total daily steps walked
Day 1	
Day 2	
Day 3	

My average daily baseline (add the numbers above up and divide by three) is: _____

My step rate

In sixty seconds I walked _____ steps.

Walkactive Steps Per Minute

If you take a hundred steps per minute for thirty minutes (so that's 3000 steps) you are doing a moderately intense form of exercise – this is ideal for overall health. Once you have mastered the basics of Walkactive – even by the end of your first session – you should find your posture pace is around 110–115 steps per minute. In other words, Walkactive is making your body work harder!

HOW ACTIVE ARE YOU REALLY?

Your average daily baseline puts you in a particular 'bracket' of activity as defined by movement scientists as follows:

- **sedentary**: fewer than 5000 steps per day (this is what you'd do just moving around the house)
- **low active**: 5000–7499 steps per day (about forty to sixty minutes, or about 2.5–3.5 miles/4–5.6km) throughout the day if you're walking at 115 steps per minute
- **somewhat active**: 7500–9999 steps per day (this is about sixty to eighty minutes or 3.5–5 miles/5.6–8km) walking per day if you are walking at 115 steps per minute
- **active**: 10,000 steps per day (this means about one hour and twenty minutes or about 5 miles/8km walking per day); unless you do a job that requires walking all day, you're most likely to achieve this by a walk of around half an hour at a fast pace (a Pace Walk), plus the steps you'd normally walk in the course of your daily activities. These will be at your 'posture pace' (the pace you use when you are keeping up your technique, but not walking fast – for instance, walking around at work).

See my tips on pages 83–5 for how to increase your daily steps.

WALKACTIVE AND DAILY STEPS: THE SCIENCE

I have found that a goal of consistently achieving 7500 steps per day is much more achievable and sustainable than 10,000 steps, which can be a real stretch for many people. But Walkactive is so much more effective than 'ordinary' walking in that 7500 Walkactive steps is easily the equivalent of 10,000 normal 'walk wrong' steps.

On average, 2000–2500 steps are equivalent to about a mile (1.6km). Walking 1 mile burns about 80 calories for a 150-pound (68kg) person. With Walkactive, you burn more calories per mile because your body is working more effectively. According to the American College of Sports Medicine, if you are doing vigorous-intensity exercise (as you are with Walkactive), then 10,000 Walkactive steps per day may be *more* than you need to do in order to be very active. If you:

- **add just 2000 steps per day** to your regular activities, you may never gain another pound (0.5kg), according to one study from the University of Colorado
- **take 6000 steps per day, you'll live longer** – sedentary people tend to move only 2000–3000 steps per day, while studies show that moving 6000 steps per day significantly improves life expectancy

- **aim for 10,000 steps, you'll lose weight** – studies show that walking around 8000–10,000 steps per day promotes weight loss
- **move 7500 Walkactive steps per day,** and you'll see the inches drop from your waistline.

CHOOSE YOUR GOAL

Right now, you probably want me to tell you how far you have to walk, or for how many minutes, in order to get 'results'. But to answer this, we first have to establish what results you want to see.

CASE STUDY: REBECCA – A FASTER-PACED LIFE

Rebecca, aged forty, started Walkactive in May 2012. She hadn't done much exercise in a while because of knee and hip injuries and she'd put on some weight. In the past she'd tried all sorts of exercise regimes, but had stuck with nothing. Now, she felt inactive and quite unconfident, and hardly ever walked anywhere. 'At first I wasn't quite sure about the Walkactive technique, and whether I'd ever be able to master it. It seemed like a lot to take on – open ankles, feel your toes spread, lift off your hips – and I hadn't even got to the arm movement yet! To be honest, it did take me a few lessons to get the hang of it. But now, I feel I really have mastered the technique.'

Because Walkactive puts less strain on joints, Rebecca is able to exercise without pain for the first time and she loves it. She also picks up tips from the people she meets at Walkactive events – she now leaves her car and walks to places in London, far more often than she ever did. And she is noticing the difference. In six months Rebecca has lost 15 inches (38cm) and 26lb (12kg) and has dropped two dress sizes. Already beautiful, Rebecca now looks incredible.

'Joanna has inspired me to make a change in my lifestyle,' says Rebecca. 'By being more active I feel and look so much better!'

Because Walkactive puts less strain on joints, Rebecca is able to exercise without pain for the first time

When people start an exercise plan they generally assume that they will get fitter, healthier and either lose weight or maintain a healthy weight. You can achieve fitness, improved health and inch loss with Walkactive, but exactly how much you have to do to reach each of these goals will depend on many factors.

The fact is, our bodies need to do different things for general health, cardiovascular fitness and weight loss or maintenance. This is why it's a good idea to think a bit about your priorities, i.e. which outcome do you care about the most? You can then target your Walkactive plan towards that specific goal.

Your health

What is health? This is not as silly a question as it may sound. You may want to be 'healthier', but what does this really mean? Many people think of health as the absence of illness, but health is defined by the World Health Organization as a state of complete physical, mental and social well-being, and not merely the absence of disease or infirmity. Walking is beneficial on both these counts: regular walking has been shown to lower your chances of common lifestyle diseases such as diabetes, heart disease and cancer – *and* it contributes to general well-being, giving you more energy and improving mood. With Walkactive you'll also lose inches as you walk for health, as your body will become so much more toned working from the inside out.

Physical fitness

There are many ways to define physical fitness, but in essence, fitness comes down to three things: endurance, balance and flexibility. Endurance is the stamina of your heart and lungs and the strength of your muscles – their ability to continue working. With improved endurance you get more energy, a spring in your step and you are able to keep going for longer. Balance and flexibility are about your body's range of motion. Without a good range of motion, you are more prone to injury and everyday activities such as reaching for the top shelf, tying up your shoe laces or undoing the back buttons of a dress can become frustratingly challenging. If you don't have good balance you are also more likely to fall. In fact, balance is often overlooked when people talk about fitness, but it does become increasingly important as we get older.

If you follow my 'Walkactive for Fitness' plan (see Chapter Six), you will see improvements in cardiovascular fitness as well as muscle strength and balance. How fast and how much your fitness level changes will depend on you: your starting point, your fitness goals and your motivation.

(TIP)   *Think inches or centimetres not weight*

I prefer to think in terms of inch loss, rather than weight loss. You're no doubt already aware that muscles weigh more than fat. This means you can tone your muscles with Walkactive, reducing fat significantly and losing lots of inches, but not necessarily drop significant amounts of weight. You'll get the body transformation you long for because of Walkactive's unique lengthening and internal tightening effect. And you'll look slimmer and more elegant as your muscles shrink-wrap themselves around your new internal framework (and yes, you can fit into those skinny jeans, dropping inches and toning up spectacularly). But the scales might not show a dramatic change. My Walkactive for Inch-Loss Plan (Chapter Seven) will show you how to transform your body in this way. Again, the speed and extent of this will depend on factors such as your motivation, starting point, diet and goals.

Inch loss

People often assume that as soon as they start to exercise they will get slim. However, exercise does not automatically do this. Evidence suggests that if you start walking 5000 steps each day your overall health will definitely improve, but whether this will also make you slim down will depend on your starting point. If you are extremely overweight, and not used to activity, then you may see very rapid inch loss at this level. But if you are already quite fit, and do not have much weight to lose, you will get healthier and more toned, but you will have to look at doing a combination of Pace Walks and building your steps up to see significant inch loss (you may have to walk up to 10,000 steps per day plus Pace Walks to see results). What you eat, of course, will also play a part in whether you lose inches.

WHAT'S IMPORTANT TO *YOU*?

Better health, improved fitness and inch loss are all great things, but do ask yourself which of these is the most important to you. Do you simply want to look lean and toned? Or are you more concerned about your health and weight – perhaps there's a history of heart disease in your family, or cancer, and you are keen to build a strong foundation in order to safeguard your body as much as you can? Or are you a new mum who wants to get toned again? Do you want more stamina – if you have a young, growing family maybe what you need most is bags of energy, so you can keep up with them as they grow? Or do you want to improve your fitness, so your athletic performance skyrockets? It's important to realise that you don't have to achieve all these goals at the same time. If you work out what your top priority is then you will stand a far greater chance of success.

For what it's worth, to my mind, the absolute best place to start is your health. Yes, I can give you a fabulous-looking bottom and I can most definitely take inches off your waistline, but it's no good looking fabulous if your cholesterol level is dangerously high or if you develop diabetes. What really matters above all else is your health. And clients who take health as their main goal often do end up seeing amazing inch loss and improved fitness levels too. And best of all, they do this without worry or struggle.

SELECT YOUR PLAN – AND STICK WITH IT

I'm now going to give you a clear sense of what you will have to do to reach your personal goal. If you choose a plan and follow my steps, you *will* see the amazing body transformation results you long for. What follows is a basic guide – I will explain each goal in far more detail in the coming chapters – but it will give you a sense of what you'll need to do.

1. Walkactive for overall health

- Achieve a baseline of 5000 steps every day, walking at 115 steps per minute.
- Follow my healthy eating guidelines (see pages 145–52).

2. Walkactive for improved fitness

- Achieve a baseline of 5000 steps every day, walking at 115 steps per minute. PLUS
- Do three Pace Walks per week, where you are walking at your OWP.

3. Walkactive for inch loss

- Achieve a baseline of 7500 steps every day, walking at 115 steps per minute. PLUS
- Do four Pace Walks at your OWP.
- Follow my Carb Curfew and other healthy eating strategies in Chapter Seven.

Once you reach your target weight it's all about weight maintenance and in order to keep your new-found figure you'll need to:

- Maintain your daily 7500 steps at 115 steps per minute. PLUS
- Do three Pace Walks per week at your OWP.
- Continue to follow my healthy eating suggestions (see pages 145–52), practising the Carb Curfew regularly.

Pace Walks: how long do you have to walk for?

When you start out, by far the most important thing is to be consistent and follow the plan for your specific goal – do the correct *number* of Pace Walks per week. Initially, your Pace Walks don't have to last very long – as little as five minutes (though with warming-up and cooling-down time, this will mean that you are actually out for twelve minutes – see page 120 for how to do this).

By far the most important thing is to do them regularly. If you skip Walkactive during the week, then try to make up for lost time by doing a mega walk at the weekend, you simply will not be doing enough to transform your body. As I said, what matters is doing the right number of Pace Walks for your goal. As your fitness improves, you'll slowly increase the duration of your Pace Walks and you'll find ways to fit them into your life, I promise.

Ultimately, you may end up with Pace Walks that last for as long as thirty to sixty minutes (including the warm-up/cool-down). If you think this sounds impossible in addition to all the steps you'll have to take, don't panic. For now, just think in terms of getting out there for a Pace Walk, the right number of times per week.

TROUBLESHOOTING

'Help! My baseline is nowhere near my daily target!' Once you've seen what your number of daily steps should be, you might be a little shocked. You may find that what you actually do is nowhere near what the daily minimum should be. If this is the case, do *not* panic – and *do not* give up! As I pointed out previously, this is about being consistent. So here's what you do to up your daily steps:

- You are going to walk for your average daily baseline, *plus* an extra 500 steps (using a good Walkactive technique, 500 steps will only take you about *five minutes*), and you're going to do this for the next seven days.
- At the start of the second week, your target is to add on yet another 500 steps. In other words, you're now walking your average baseline *plus 1000 steps* for the next seven days.
- Repeat this, adding an extra 500 steps every week, until you reach your daily target.
- I think it's also useful to think in five-minute 'slots' – the time it takes to make a cup of tea; four slots of five minutes sounds far less intimidating than saying you have to walk an extra twenty minutes every day.

MAKE WALKACTIVE WORK FOR YOU

Sometimes the practicalities seem to get in the way of the best intentions – lack of time, weather conditions or even the wrong shoes, to name a few. I'm going to show you how to deal with such practicalities, so that you can fit Walkactive into your life whatever's happening.

Coping with time restrictions

If you think you'll struggle to find time to build up your daily steps, there are many ways you can deal with this. Here are some tricks to start with:

- **Plot routes** Find a five-minute, ten-minute and fifteen-minute route from your home, your work, the school gates, the bus stop or anywhere that is a regular part of your day. That way, when you have a spare moment or time to walk, you'll be ready to Walkactive without wondering 'Where shall I go?'

- **Piggy-back on a daily habit** Find something that you do every day – whether it's brushing your teeth or buying your daily paper, checking your emails or opening your purse to buy your lunchtime sandwich. Whatever you choose, decide to put a certain number of steps on your pedometer before you

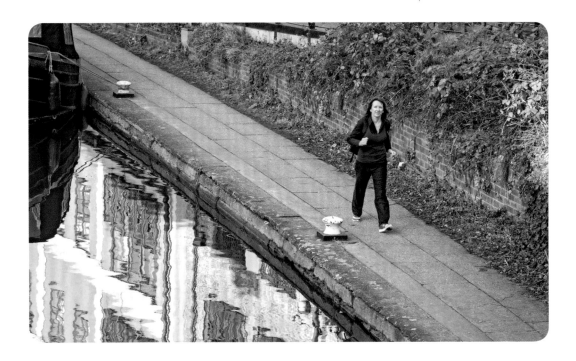

do it. For instance, you could walk a longer route, rather than the most direct one when going to buy the paper, go up and down the stairs six times while brushing your teeth or walk round the block before checking your emails. Whatever it is, make this your rule: 'Add steps before I do it.'

- **Split your day into zones** Trying to do all your steps in one go can be a huge challenge. It can help to split your day into four-hour 'zones' and aim to complete 1000 steps in each one. For example, 7–11am, 11–3pm, 3–7pm and 7pm–bedtime. If you do this, then you'll come to the end of each day with at least 4000 steps accumulated. Your other daily activities will push you over your health-criteria threshold, and you'll make it to 5000.

- **Whenever possible, walk and talk** Instead of sitting down to make phone calls, resolve to walk and talk wherever you can – even if it is just pacing around your office or house while you talk. This can be even more effective if you and someone else agree not to talk on the phone (or even exchange texts or emails) at all until you are physically together – that way you'll have a lot of information to exchange as you walk. This works particularly well with parents after a school drop-off or work colleagues during lunch breaks.

- **Make walking part of your life** Instead of imposing 'duty' sessions where you have to go out and Walkactive, think about Walkactive becoming part of your life – weave it into your daily activities and routines. You're trying to make movement the norm, rather than an activity you squeeze in at the end of the day.

- **Play games in the park** This is especially great if you have kids. Set two-minute time tests where you take it in turns to see who records the most steps in that time (obviously, you will be using a perfect Walkactive technique, but your kids can be running). Log the steps and repeat five times to see if you can improve. You can also get the kids to see how far you can walk in two minutes, using trees or benches as markers.

- **Set your alarm earlier – and do it!** Even twenty minutes helps. This sounds obvious, but it's so worth it – especially as pre-breakfast you'll be burning into your fat reserves as an energy source.

- **Tweak your activities** Little changes in your routine can add up to a mile or two per day. Here are some things you can try:
  - Park further from your destination.
  - Take the stairs rather than the lift or escalator.
  - March on the spot for one minute every hour.

'I've been doing Walkactive for a year now. I went on a residential programme and have been doing the courses ever since – my fitness, skin and posture are all so much better. I used to be very stiff in my shoulders and now the mobility in my neck, shoulders and upper back is just so much better. I've fitted it into my life by getting most of my Walkactive steps done in the morning after I have dropped the children at school. I still work, so it's not as if I have loads of time to spare, but I find planning in this Walkactive time early in the day is vital. I've made three routes back from school that I use according to the time I have that day. On a good day I can get 4000 steps under my belt before work. Even if I can only spare ten minutes – I make it sacrosanct. If I get those steps on my pedometer before work, then I feel getting to 7500 by the end of the day is doable.'

YASMIN, 38, WALKACTIVE CLUB MEMBER

– Walk up and down the stairs or round the sofa during TV ad breaks.
– Work out the number of steps your normal routes take – say, to the corner shop, school gates or train station – then change them to find ones that add on, say, 500–1000 steps. If you're worried about time, don't be – with the Walkactive technique, using your accelerators, you'll be going a lot faster so you will still save time.
– Do your Abdominal Js while waiting for traffic lights to change, when crossing the road or waiting for the kettle to boil. Make it a habit.
– If you work in an office get into the habit of doing two of three circuits of the office before you make a cup of tea or coffee.

 TIP *Don't forget about posture pace*

In your day-to-day life, when you are accumulating your steps and using your Walkactive technique, you are likely to be mostly walking at your posture pace (see page 65). This is where you are being true to your Walkactive technique without focusing intensely on it or using your accelerators. You'll use posture pace as you walk around a supermarket, or walk to a meeting with colleagues. Don't overlook posture pace: you might not be increasing your fitness when you walk this way (it doesn't give you the cardiovascular benefits of a Pace Walk), but it works miracles on transforming your body: you are correcting your posture and joint alignment and toning your muscles with every single step. Posture pace makes a radical difference to your body shape.

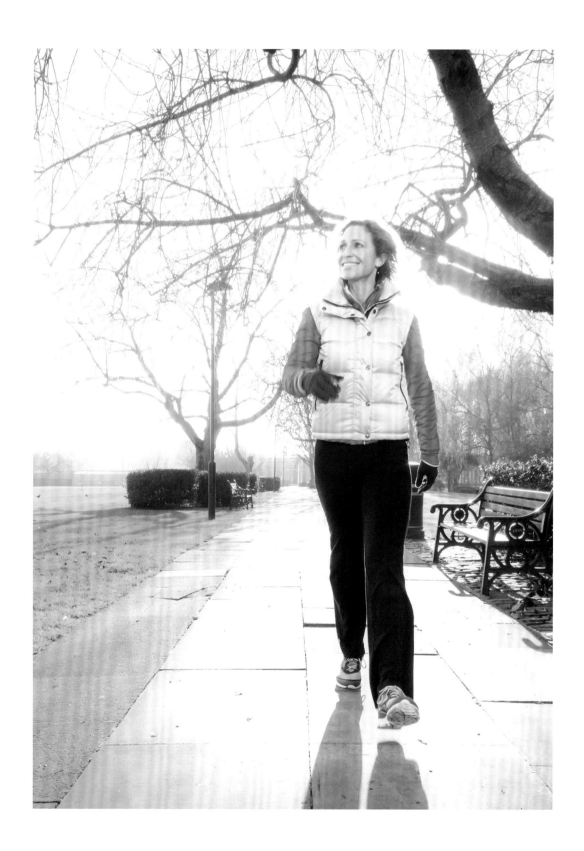

Facing the elements

Walkactive is becoming part of your life and this means you do it regardless of the weather. It's a bit like waiting for the perfect calm week – if you wait for the right weather (at least in the UK) you'll only go out about twice a year! To make Walkactive a real part of who you are, it needs to be comfortable, practical and to feel good – whatever the weather. If you are boiling hot or freezing cold, bundled up so you can't move your arms or blinded by the sun, Walkactive is not going to be fun, and your technique will be compromised. But if you are wearing the right things, you'll be comfortable, so making Walkactive much more manageable, regardless of the weather. Use the folowing guide as a way to address comfort in general – you may well not be able to dress like this in the office or if you're walking to a party, but you can adapt your work or going-out clothes as necessary if you've given it some thought.

Cold, crisp, dry weather

Think thin, fitted layers, rather than anything big, bulky or baggy. You do need to keep warm, but if you're layered up like the Michelin man it will be far harder to appreciate how your body is moving. This will throw out your postural alignment and get in the way of your technique. So wear several thin layers, rather than one or two thicker ones.

Top half

- Wear a base layer of a technical fabric T-shirt that is close fitting so that your other layers fit smoothly over the top. Cotton may be natural, but when you sweat the moisture stays close to your skin, and when it cools down can leave you feeling cold. Technical fabrics, on the other hand, are made to draw sweat away from your body, so they keep you at a more stable, comfortable temperature.
- Wear a lightweight long-sleeved layer over the top of your base layer.
- A fitted, lightweight technical fabric full-zip jacket is great over that – a full-length zip makes it easy to remove or just undo a little as you get warm.
- You may want a sleeveless fleece gilet for extra warmth; this is optional, depending on the temperature.
- A shell jacket with a full-length zip is also useful – again, you can undo it for temperature control.

Bottom half

- Stretch exercise trousers or running-style trousers are ideal – not too baggy though or they'll get in the way.
- You can add another layer underneath, if it is particularly cold. It's important to keep your legs and ankles warm to keep them mobile, and to help your body's circulation (so that you don't strain your muscles).

- Bamboo fabric socks are particularly comfortable and feel like you are wearing cashmere – I'd recommend wearing two pairs of these, rather than one thicker pair. Go for ankle or knee-length (rather than trainer-style) socks to help keep your ankles warm.

Extremities and accessories

- Hands: go for gloves with a longer wrist section so that your forearms stay warm too; this will improve the temperature of the blood and will therefore keep your hands warmer than gloves that stop at the wrist.
- Neck and head: consider a snood made from a technical thermal fleece. You can move it off your head if you get too warm – and some lift up over your mouth and nose in cold conditions. Thermal fleece fabric is good for comfort as it helps to regulate body temperature, locking in the heat, while pulling sweat away from the skin.
- Ankle or leg warmers: these keep ankles warm and flexible so they 'open' well with each step. I'd strongly advise these if you're feeling discomfort down the front of your leg or if your circulation isn't great. I'm not talking about ballet-style leg warmers – the ones I mean are more like compression warming socks that go all the way to the knee. The other advantage of these is that you can remove them easily if you get too warm or roll them down.

 TIP *Layer up after a Pace Walk in cold weather*

After you have finished a Pace Walk it's important to have another layer to put on. You may not be feeling cold while you are walking fast, but it's easy to get uncomfortably chilled as you cool down. So as you get warm, take one of your layers off, but keep it with you, ready to put on when you finish the Pace Walk.

Glow in the dark

Safety should always be your number-one priority and in the winter months you're likely to be walking in the dark a lot. So look for kit with reflective straps and strips or invest in some reflective bands that you can put on whatever you're wearing. You can also get lights that fit on a backpack, if you are walking to and from work.

Cold, wet weather

Again, think lots of thin layers to keep you warm without adding bulk. And, of course, you'll need to wear really effective waterproofs that breathe, so you don't get hot and sweaty.

Top half

Think thin layers as above, but with a technical waterproof jacket that allows your skin to breathe. This means that your warmth can evaporate, rather than stay close to your skin where it will cool down, leaving you feeling chilled afterwards.

Bottom half

Waterproof trousers are useful; don't panic, you don't have to wear really baggy old-fashioned ones – many good sports companies have stylish and practical pairs and golf clothing companies are also worth investigating. Good waterproof trousers will be expensive – but worth it if you are going to be out in the elements.

Extremities

I'd recommend waterproof or water-resistant gloves (as full waterproof gloves are hard to find) and a waterproof jacket with a hood. If you don't like a hood too close to your face, wear a baseball cap underneath. I personally favour a baseball cap. The peak will keep the drizzle out of your eyes, allowing you to keep your correct eye line and not drop your head down to keep the rain out of your face. Doing this will only compromise the fab symmetry we have created through the upper torso!

Warm, balmy or hot weather

It can be hard to know what to wear if the sun is going in and out and it could get really hot or cool down completely. The basic principle is to give yourself options. So – once again – layers are the key.

Top half

- You want to wear T-shirts that will stop you either overheating or getting cold if the sun goes in. Choose technical fabrics designed for exercise that will allow your skin to breathe and therefore stop you feeling hot and sweaty.
- Have one or two light layers with you, so you can adjust to whatever the sun is – or isn't – doing. You can put discarded layers in a backpack or tie them around your waist. The main thing is to keep your arms free.
- Wear sunscreen! Burning skin is not a good feeling – and, of course, sun damage can cause skin cancer.

Bottom half

- Three-quarter-/knee-length trousers – if you are not a fan of shorts, but trousers are too hot, three-quarter or knee-length trousers can be a more flattering way to stay cool. Choose a fabric that lets you move and allows your skin to breathe. I'm a really big fan of three-quarter-length trousers in most weathers, actually – if the ground is wet, you don't end up with soggy trouser cuffs that drape on your trainers, getting your feet wet.
- A pair of Lycra shorts under a short tennis-style skirt can be flattering for women, while for men another option is a pair of lighter-weight shorts that have a technical component to let your skin breathe.

TIP ....
Avoid warm-weather chafing

Chafing – where areas of your skin rub together – can be a real problem in warm weather. Pre-empt this by applying a small amount of a natural sports lubricant (like Vaseline, only better) on delicate, vulnerable areas – between your arms and chest or between the inner thighs. Once the skin is broken it can be very painful and will limit the intensity of your Walkactive sessions – so prevention is best.

General kit

The right basic kit will allow your body to move in the right way, so you keep true to your Walkactive technique. It will also make you more comfortable – so you'll want to do it more.

In addition to your trusty pedometer and weather-appropriate clothes (see above), you will need the following.

Shoes

With your Walkactive technique your foot will become a lot more mobile. Dig out your trainers or walking shoes and check that the soles are not too thick. Stiff soles, particularly in mountain-style walking boots, can make it much harder to keep an active foot and to feel how your foot spreads. Shoes that are too narrow will also stop your foot from spreading. A lighter-weight, thinner-soled more flexible training shoe with a wider toe box (such as 'barefoot' shoes) is preferable because your toes will spread as you master Walkactive.

Get into the habit of keeping your lightweight Walkactive trainers with you. This way, when you are walking any distance, you can swap your day-to-day shoes for your Walkactive ones, rather than walk in restrictive or heeled work shoes.

A baseball cap

This will keep both rain and sun out of your eyes – this is important because stooping or squinting affect your posture, getting in the way of your shoulder, neck and upper-back alignment.

A backpack

Try to switch from a shoulder bag to a backpack – as Walkactive becomes part of your day, you might need to carry more things (for instance, to work). A shoulder bag will affect your posture, whereas a backpack will allow you to Walkactive. Opt for a backpack with a chest strap so that your arms can swing, your shoulders can be in the correct position and your spine can rotate as it should. If your backpack doesn't have a front strap, it is possible that when you draw your shoulders back, the arm straps will keep slipping off. You will then 'lock' your shoulders and stop using your arms properly. Your back then becomes rigid and your Walkactive technique is compromised. You can customise an existing backpack if you don't want to buy a new one – just tie a simple piece of string between the straps drawing them closer together at your chest. If, at any time, you do have to carry a shoulder bag, try to wear it across your body, rather than over just one shoulder.

 ┄┄┄┄┄┄┄┄┄┄┄┄┄┄┄┄┄┄┄┄┄┄

Handbags and heels

- **Handbags** *If you are carrying a handbag, it's better to have one with a longer shoulder strap that you can wear across the body ('messenger style'), rather than one you wear over one shoulder. Carrying a bag over one shoulder – particularly if it's heavy – will stop your spine from being symmetrically aligned. This will get in the way of the correct Walkactive posture (and, eventually, cause you back problems).*
- **Heels** *I'm often asked, 'But what do you do when you are wearing heels – surely you can't do Walkactive?' Well you may not achieve a fully active foot and open ankle, but you can still be focused on your hip lift and shoulder alignment – in fact, by mastering Walkactive many of my clients have found they walk better in their heels than they used to!*

A waist bag

Waist bags or bum bags can be useful when you are going out specifically to do a Pace or Technique Walk and only need to take a few essentials, such as your keys and a phone. Go for a snug, streamlined design, and wear it in the small of your back, rather than at the front where it can get in the way of your technique. A waist bag that is designed to hold a water bottle is great too – ideally, go for one that incorporates the bottle itself which should sit neatly within the bag, rather than dangling down. Basically, you want to keep everything neat and streamlined, so that you can focus on your body without the distraction or discomfort of annoying flaps or straps.

TROUBLESHOOTING

Here are some common problems or concerns clients often have at first, when they're 'just doing it'. I'm going to show you how to tackle these so they don't get in your way.

'I feel silly walking through town waving my arms!' This is very common – you're changing the way you move and it's bound to feel odd. On my residential programmes and training camps I often do what I call the 'Active Passive Drill'. It's best to do this once you've completed three or four Technique Walks and a couple of Pace Walks, so everything doesn't feel too alien. Here's what you do:

- Find yourself a stretch of reflective shop windows or a friend who can give you feedback. You are going to walk a short distance – probably 25–50 metres – and the first time, you're going to walk it wrong – as you used to walk: think passive foot, sitting into your hips, closed off ankle. Notice how this makes your body feel and move and how laboured and clunky your movements are. Look at your reflection or get your friend to give you feedback on how you look.
- Now, repeat the same distance, but this time put all your Walkactive technique into place – your open ankle, your active foot, lifting out of your hips. Feel and see the difference.

When I do this drill at my Walkactive events the comments are enlightening! Nobody has an interest in lying – they all tell it as they see it and when I ask the 'observer', 'So, does that person look silly doing Walkactive?' Hand on heart, 100 per cent of them reply with a resounding 'NO!' It's when you power walk and are tense or walk wrong that you look silly! (See the comments opposite.) With Walkactive you look strong and elegant. You may *feel* you look silly at first because the movement pattern is new

to you. And yes, it will feel a little awkward initially. But the more natural and embedded Walkactive becomes, the better you'll look. And people will notice!

'I get bored on long walks!' When people begin to master Walkactive two things happen: they get fab results without always having to go for long-distance walks, and they feel a natural body momentum so that, actually, they don't want to stop walking. Walkactive's natural momentum propels you forward; you feel you are working hard, but at the same time, it feels easier, and you want to do it more. It's kind of addictive. Walkactive becomes more enjoyable as you progress with it: you'll become motivated by finding yourself a new route, setting yourself time targets or step targets, listening to my audio workouts. You can also download an audio book to listen to as you walk, or you can listen to music. This can really help, but be wary of choosing music with too fast a beat as it can make you snatch your steps and shorten your stride, and you don't want to miss out on the lengthening effect of Walkactive!

'I want to walk with my wife, but she can't keep up when I walk at my Pace Walk speed and when I walk at her speed it's too slow!' OK, there are a couple of things you can do about this. Start off walking together. First, go through your technique and pay

Passive Walking vs Walkactive – What Participants *Really* Think

Here are some genuine comments from clients who've done the Active Passive Drill. Remember these are real clients, real comments – all unprompted by me!

 When you walk passively you look:

- sluggish

- older, thicker in the waist

- slumped around the shoulders

- shuffling foot movement

- your feet are really dragging and scuffing

- lazy

- less happy, depressed

- lethargic

- disengaged

- this type of walk looks silly and embarrassing!

 When you Walkactive you look:

- WOW – amazing!

- slimmer

- happier

- younger

- more agile, open and receptive

- smooth

- more upright and purposeful but flowing

- ten years younger! Your posture is so much better

- less stiff, fitter!

particular attention to your hip lift. Then after about five to eight minutes, once you are both warmed up and you've had a bit of a chat – you can do one of the following:

• **Mini 'out/back' walks**: pick up your pace, stretch out in front of her using your accelerators, walk to a certain point, then turn and walk back and have another chat; you are still doing Walkactive, but you have taken off your accelerators. Repeat several times. You get your Pace as well as your Technique Walks in one hit.

• **'Sheep dog'**: after the warm-up, you walk ahead to a distance then turn and walk back to her, but walk past her in a different direction for a short way before you turn to join her. Repeat.

• **'Hare and hound'**: this works if you're walking to a certain point, then turning round and going home. You both walk together to the point where you turn to go back – but as she turns, you keep walking in the same direction for two, three, maybe four minutes, even though she's turned to walk home. After this,

CASE STUDY: KEN – FITTING WALKACTIVE INTO A BUSY SCHEDULE

Ken, fifty-five, a record producer, hired me for one-to-one sessions after his divorce. A tall and handsome man, Ken loved parties, food and wine – and hated exercise. His waistline was really showing it, as were his posture and muscle tone. His life was full-on and hectic – a round of constant meetings, business meals and executive travel. Often, his day would consist of stepping from chauffeured car to meeting room to car to restaurant to office or on to a plane – with almost no walking. His average baseline steps came in at around 2500–3000 per day, so while he was tired at the end of the day, he was firmly in the 'sedentary' category. Ken was busy from the moment he woke up to the moment he went to sleep and he didn't see how he could possibly fit walking into his life. But together we came up with simple ways for him to increase his daily steps. His PA would only give him coffee once he'd walked around his office for at least ten minutes. He'd then keep pacing as he made his first phone calls – and then throughout the day, every time he got on the phone, Ken would walk. He'd get his chauffeur to drop him three blocks away from a meeting or restaurant, and meet him afterwards a block or two down the road.

These small changes alone doubled Ken's steps to 5000 per day. But his target was also to fit in three Pace Walks every week with me, lasting for about an hour each. Realistically, he only ever really managed one Pace Walk – for around twenty-two minutes. Still, I assured him that the main thing was to do *something* and, to his credit, he persisted. It worked! Ken took 4 inches (10cm) off his waistline and lost 9lb (4.8kg) in just six weeks. He now has more energy than he's had in years, looks much more svelte and has started dating again. He's seen other changes too. He told me he'd always sit down at parties as he was self-conscious about his height, but he noticed that after Walkactive he no longer felt the need to do this – he now stands tall, conscious of his improved posture and muscle tone. He looks and feels fabulous. 'What really astonished me,' he says, 'is how small changes can add up to such a big difference. You don't need to find extra time for Walkactive – you just need to change your habits. It really works.'

you turn and try to catch her up – still, of course, using your perfect Walkactive technique and your accelerators. This is an interesting one, as the slower walker is now the one in the lead, so is encouraged to use her accelerators too. Many people who feel they are naturally 'slower' often walk their best in this situation as the competitive instinct kicks in.

• **Perfect your Walkactive technique without your accelerators**: this is a non-pace option. You do your Abdominal Js the whole time and focus on perfecting your technique. This is a toning and posture session and will do amazing things to your body too. You can also do this when walking with someone who knows nothing about Walkactive – though you probably will feel compelled to tell them about it when you see them walking wrong!

YOU CAN DO THIS!

I know you have a complicated life, packed with demands and distractions, some of which you just can't control. But you're not the only one – and that's how I know you can do this! I've worked with thousands of people just like you whose lives are overwhelming and chock-a-block with commitments and demands. It takes planning, but my clients do find ways to make Walkactive part of their lives – and they see radical results across all aspects of their lives: they sit and stand differently; they feel better about themselves; they get 'out there' more, feel less shy and more confident, both socially and at work; they need less medication for health problems, feel less pain in joints or strains and they exude health and well-being; they drop dress sizes and their waists shrink; they do better at their job and their chosen sport. In short, they embrace life – and so can you. So don't let anything stand in your way.

It's time to just do it!

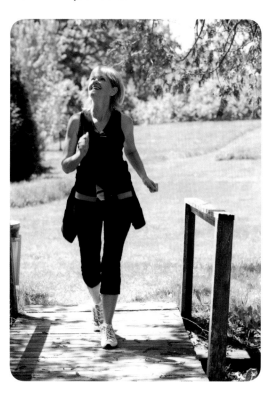

CHAPTER FIVE

WALKACTIVE FOR HEALTH

'If Walkactive came in pill form, everyone would be popping it!'

As is the case before beginning any exercise programme, it is important to talk to your doctor about your plans, particularly if you are not fighting fit. If you are battling health problems – even very serious ones – your doctor should be able to reassure you about the level of intensity that's right for you and any particular health issue, and tell you about any 'warning signs' to watch out for. It's important to have this peace of mind – and this way you can give Walkactive your best shot without worrying or holding back.

Walkactive is going to make a massive difference to your health. Outwardly, you will begin to look better within a very short time of starting your programme: your skin tone will improve, your muscles will begin to lengthen and tone up, you'll notice a whittled waist and a vastly improved posture. All this will give you the appearance of youthful vitality. But the most important work will be going on inside your body – strengthening your heart and lungs, lowering the levels of bad cholesterol in your blood, balancing blood-sugar levels and maintaining a healthy weight.

If you follow the plan I've laid out in this chapter, you will improve your ability to resist (or recover from) many

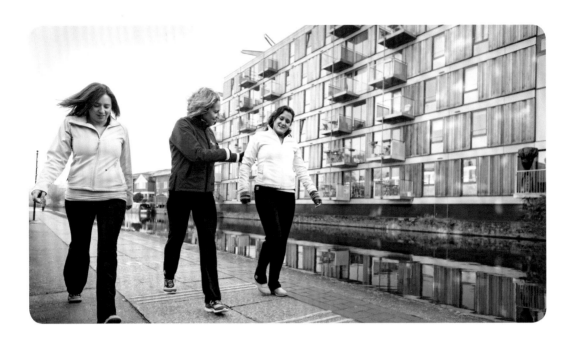

common and devastating illnesses and ailments. You will improve your chances not just of living longer, but of living with energy and a *joie de vivre* – a spring in your step. You will increase your mobility and balance and have fewer aches and pains, illnesses and injuries. All in all, Walkactive is your ticket to a healthier, happier you: your body is going to thank you for this – as will your loved ones!

 TIP *Check it out with your doctor*

As already stated, before starting any new activity, you need to check with your GP so your specific and personal condition is accommodated. But as the saying goes, 'Walk your dog every day – even if you don't have one!'

WHAT CAN WALKACTIVE DO FOR YOUR HEALTH?

There are many ways in which Walkactive can improve your health. Let's take a look at each of them in turn.

Walkactive can...

Help you live longer

There is already a large body of evidence to suggest that walking briskly each day (for thirty minutes) can improve your life expectancy. With Walkactive you do just that!

Boost cardiovascular health

Cardiovascular problems (heart disease, heart attack, stroke, heart failure) are the

UK's biggest killers, causing more than one in three of all deaths. The British Heart Foundation recommends walking as a great form of exercise for cardiovascular health, and there are many scientific studies showing the benefits to the heart of daily walking. The Honolulu Heart Study, published in 2002, looked at 8000 men and found that those who walked just 2 miles (3.2km) per day cut their risk of death from heart disease almost in half. A Danish study found that people who went on a fast daily walk (that's your Walkactive Pace Walk) halved their chance of a heart attack or stroke.

Walkactive, in short, is going to make a vast difference to your cardiovascular health.

Help you maintain a healthy weight

You can use Walkactive for inch loss (see Chapter Seven), but it is also a fabulous weight-management tool – keeping you at a healthy weight for life. Being overweight or obese is associated with so many diseases, from breast and colon cancers to diabetes and cardiovascular diseases. Many of us put on pounds as we age, but Walkactive will help you to resist 'middle-age spread' because it becomes a part of your life, for ever. In our supersize, sedentary culture this is an incredible long-term health benefit. And it's so easy!

'I have been practising the techniques more or less daily and already I am aware that I am starting to feel fitter. More importantly, I feel less pressure on my back. I used to be a keen tennis player, but had to give it up because of lower-back disc problems. This is the first form of exercise I've found that doesn't hurt my back and that I actually enjoy. At the moment, I'm still at the concentrating stage, but I am determined to progress. I feel like I've found "the answer" at last.'

KEVIN, 45, ATTENDED A ONE-DAY WALKACTIVE COURSE

Improve cancer outcomes

According to Cancer Research UK, physical activity – such as brisk walking daily – can help to prevent more than 3000 cases of cancer in the UK every year. There is so much evidence now to show that exercise such as walking can help to prevent all sorts of cancers – and Walkactive works because you build it into your life. It becomes a habit, not a fad. Walkactive can also help if you do develop cancer: studies show that daily walking can be an excellent way to improve your chances of cancer recovery and can help to tackle some of the debilitating side-effects of treatment, such as fatigue. Daily walking can also lower the chance that the cancer will come back when treatment ends. Macmillan Cancer Support is so convinced of the benefits of walking that it has implemented a national programme of 'Health Walks' for cancer recovery and prevention. Of course, the beauty of Walkactive is that you can adapt it to your body's needs and capabilities, so it really is a wonderful way to exercise both during and after serious illness.

Lower your risk of diabetes (and help to control it)

The number of people diagnosed with type-2 diabetes (mainly caused by obesity) is rising rapidly in the UK. But here's the good news: research shows that walking for thirty minutes per day will significantly lower your chances of developing type-2 diabetes (whether you are overweight now or not). A study published in 2011 on the *British Medical Journal* website also shows that if you have already been diagnosed, and walk 10,000 steps per day, you can significantly reduce the effects of your diabetes. Your 5000 Walkactive steps could therefore go a long way towards effective diabetes management.

Improve brain power and ward off dementia

Studies show that daily walking is not just good for the body; it's also good for the brain. Walkactive can help to keep your mind

Walkactive and Breast Cancer

If you have been diagnosed with or treated for breast cancer, Walkactive really is for you. Published in the *Journal of the American Medical Association* in 2005, a large study from Harvard University found that women who walked three to five hours per week dramatically reduced their risk of death from cancer – that's just thirty minutes of Walkactive per day. You may have to build up slowly to this target, but Walkactive allows you to do just that: it works *with* your body, not against it.

sharp and could ward off dementia. A study of older people, published in 2012 in the American Heart Association journal *Stroke*, found that those who did regular physical activity, such as walking, reduced their risk of vascular-related dementia by 40 per cent and their risk of cognitive impairment (your thinking, knowing and remembering skills) by a massive 60 per cent. These really are significant, persuasive findings – surely enough to get you out there walking as you age gracefully!

Boost your mood

There is a great deal of evidence to show that walking not only improves mood and enhances well-being (partly because when you exercise your body releases endorphins – so-called 'feelgood' chemicals), but that it

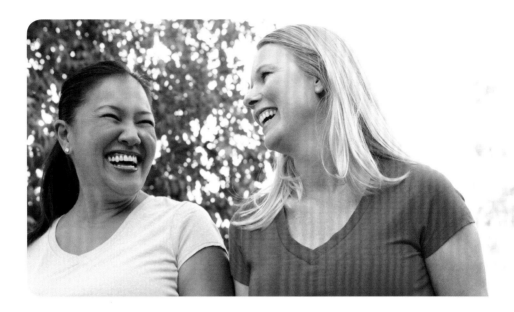

may also be a great way to treat depression. In fact, some research shows that walking may work as well as anti depressant medication in treating depression.

'I'm a teacher and educational consultant and was on anti depressants for eight years – I tried everything – alternative therapies, exercise classes – but nothing changed my dependency on the medication to help me feel better. Until I tried Walkactive. I've now been off the medication for two years, during which I've gone through redundancy and several stressful family changes, but Walkactive has kept me feeling positive and, most importantly, off the medication. This is the best I've felt in years.'

CLAUDIA, 64, WALKACTIVE MEMBER

Help with stress and anxiety management

Exercise has also been shown to help with stress and anxiety. Daily walking allows your body to let go of physical tension and has those wonderful mood-boosting effects mentioned earlier. All in all, Walkactive could change the way you see the world!

Prevent erectile dysfunction

There is some evidence to show that sedentary men can reduce the risk of erectile dysfunction by daily exercise equivalent to walking briskly for 2 miles (3.2km). Men can delay erectile issues by ten years if they do this. So guys, there's one excellent reason to build Walkactive into your day from mid-life onwards!

CASE STUDY: SANDY – METABOLIC SYNDROME

Sandy, fifty-five, is a copywriter who spends all day at her desk at home. 'I literally fall out of bed and slide on to my office chair,' she says. 'When Joanna asked me to record my daily steps with a pedometer, I knew it would be low, but I was not prepared for it to be as low as it was! I recorded 1836 on day one, 2213 on day two and 1654 on day three. I did slightly freak at that point.'

Sandy is overweight and has to take medication for a cluster of conditions that her GP calls 'metabolic syndrome'. I set Sandy the goal of increasing her daily steps to 5000 – the baseline for healthy benefits. 'I hate exercise and I am naturally lazy,' she says. While she didn't reach a consistent daily total of 5000 plus, Sandy did make an average of about 4500 steps per day. I encouraged her to reach for the 5000, but reassured her that 4500 was a huge improvement on her starting point. And it worked. After she had been doing Walkactive for a few months, Sandy went to see her GP, who was able to reduce her medication for both blood pressure and high cholesterol.

'This was such a positive step for me,' she says. 'I did feel better physically, and I know I could probably feel even better if I did more. But the most important thing was that I could do this without going completely out of my comfort zone. I am in control now and the fact that my GP has reduced my medication is a huge confidence boost. My balance is better as well as I'm using my feet more effectively – I'm no longer shuffling around; I have a spring in my step and this is making me feel like I'd like to do more. I can't deny that I'm still a naturally lazy person, but I now know that Walkactive works – I've seen the concrete, unarguable results in my blood pressure and cholesterol levels. I feel like I have more control over my health for the first time – and believe me, that's a great feeling.'

How Sandy increased her steps

- She stopped using the bathroom on the same floor as her workspace.
- She set pedometer targets every two hours – with a reminder note on her desk.
- She did the steps, even if it meant just pacing on the spot after each small project was completed at her desk.
- She made herself do 2000 steps before lunch every day.

CASE STUDY: STAN – RECLAIMING MOBILITY

Stan, a gentleman in his late seventies, came to listen to me talk while I was giving a lecture series on board the luxury cruise liner *Azura*, with over 3000 passengers and 2000 crew. I gave six lectures in two weeks to a varied audience – people of all ages and fitness and motivation levels.

Even though the auditorium was always crowded, I was aware of Stan from the outset. He was unstable, walked with a stick and needed some help to get seated. His balance was not that great, partly because he walked with a passive shuffle, and partly because I could see that he was becoming more and more dependent on his stick, so he wasn't using his stabilising abdominal muscles. His posture was seriously compromised. This was not only causing back pain, it was catapulting him towards losing his physical independence. As I talked, I hoped that my words would somehow reach Stan and give him the confidence to try the technique.

At the end of my sixth lecture I held an open-forum session, taking questions from the audience. Just as I was drawing the session to a close, Stan's hand went up. He asked if he could share his story. Of course, I was keen to hear more. I'd noticed that Stan was moving decidedly more easily by this sixth lecture and I wanted to know how he felt.

Stan explained that after my first talk, when I'd introduced Walkactive and gone through the four-part technique, he had gone straight out on to the promenade deck and given it a go – paying particular attention to his feet. He'd concentrated on moving from a passive to an active foot, and on building an awareness in his hips – lifting out of the hips rather than sitting into them. On that very first day Stan had only been able to walk around a quarter of the promenade deck before he had to stop – that's equivalent to approximately 500 small steps.

He then explained to the audience, who were listening intently now, that he had been practising Walkactive every day since, focusing on feet, hips and – though this was very hard for him – his neck and shoulder position. After twelve days, he could now walk two whole laps of the promenade deck – without his stick!

continued

As he told his story I could feel the joy filling up the room. Everyone was rooting for Stan. He was so grateful – and so amazed at what his body could do. When he'd finished, other people started to comment. They said how different he looked, how amazed they were by his achievement. Others said they'd noticed a difference in their own posture and pace too.

I was so very moved by this man's story, and by the audience's reaction to it. Of course, I absolutely love the fact that Walkactive will give you a pert bottom and take inches off your waistline. But if you are struggling with your balance and physical confidence, and rapidly losing your independence, the fact that Walkactive gives you your health and independence back – well, that feels incredibly powerful to me. Stan is what Walkactive is all about. Stan is why I love what I do.

INVEST IN YOUR FUTURE

If you spend just thirty minutes walking every day that adds up to just ninety-one days over the next twelve years of your life. Since you can add years to your life by daily walking, this is surely an amazing time payoff! Think about it this way – you'd invest in your family's future or in your pension without a second thought. Doesn't it make sense to invest in your health?

If you wait until you actually develop a health problem, you will almost certainly spend more than thirty minutes per day on taking medication, undergoing surgery, treatments and recovery, getting yourself to and from appointments and dealing with finances. And if you are reluctant to do Walkactive because you 'hate exercise', imagine how much more you will hate surgery, treatments and all the bottles of pills you'll have to take as you develop health problems? Surely it makes sense to invest just thirty minutes per day in Walkactive instead – it's far more productive and enjoyable than being unwell.

So do it *now* – don't wait.

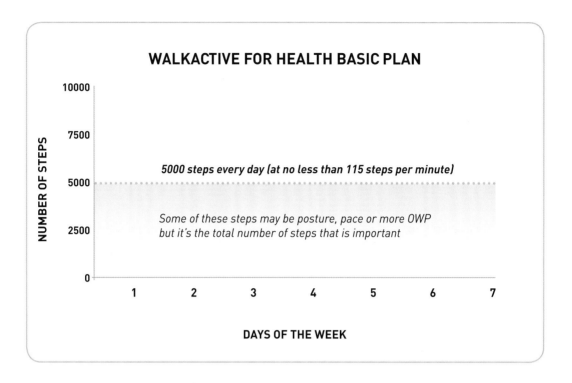

WALKACTIVE FOR HEALTH BASIC PLAN

5000 steps every day (at no less than 115 steps per minute)

Some of these steps may be posture, pace or more OWP but it's the total number of steps that is important

NUMBER OF STEPS

DAYS OF THE WEEK

WALKACTIVE FOR HEALTH: WHAT YOU NEED TO DO

It's very simple – just follow the Walkactive for Health Rules:

- **Walk 5000 Walkactive steps every day.** Yes, every single day, seven days per week. That's the most important thing.
- **Be consistent.** I cannot stress this enough. There may be a day or two per week where you don't make it to 5000, but *try* to do it every day.
- **Focus on your technique.** A faster pace is good, so yes, do try to walk at your Optimum Walking Pace (OWP) when you can, but

some of your steps will be at your posture pace, and that's fine. By mastering and consistently using the Walkactive technique you will go over the critical threshold of 115 steps per minute. This is what matters. Your posture, mobility and shape will all change too, even when you are not at your OWP.

The dos and don'ts of Walkactive for health

- **Do** little and often – that's what counts.
- **Don't** do nothing on Monday, Tuesday and Wednesday and think you can do loads the rest of the week to make up for it – this is a completely false economy.

- **Do** look for opportunities within your daily routine to increase your steps.
- **Don't** try to do it all in one big walk per day. You're likely to find this hard to maintain. As you get better you can build up the number of minutes you walk in a continual block (maybe try three lots of ten minutes or six lots of five). But if you think in terms of doing your 5000 steps per day in one go, you could find it too much of a burden.
- **Do** get some steps under your belt as early in the day as possible – this will make your target feel so much more manageable.
- **Don't** leave it later and later in the day: you'll start to feel pressurised and that could make it too challenging.
- **Don't** fall into the trap of thinking that because you are busy you are being physically active.
- **Do** wear your pedometer to record your steps. Perception and reality can be very different! Make building your baseline number of steps your priority.
- **Don't** forget to use your technique.
- **Do** remember it's the quality that is important – trust my Walkactive technique: it works.
- **Don't** think that because many of the benefits aren't obviously visible (for instance, effects on blood pressure or cholesterol levels, or cancer prevention) they aren't there. Some of the most important changes going on in your body because of Walkactive may be invisible, but they *are* happening. And they matter – a lot.
- **Do** remind yourself of all the amazing, scientifically documented preventative and health-giving benefits of walking daily (see pages 97–100).

'I've been doing Walkactive for almost a year now, and I hardly recognise myself. I'm off the anti depressants, my doctor says my bad cholesterol levels have gone down, and I am almost two stone [12.6kg] lighter. I've built Walkactive into my commute, I walk every lunch hour, and I walk after dinner every evening to wind down. I almost never get sick, I have 100 per cent more energy, and I'm happier than I've been in a long while. If Walkactive came in pill form everyone would be popping it.'

JIM, 49, ATTENDED ONE-DAY WALKACTIVE WORKSHOP

NAVIGATING THE 24

If you are struggling with the idea of finding time for Walkactive – and if the health benefits I've outlined aren't enough to motivate you, try looking at your time in a different way.

Think of it like this: there are twenty-four hours in the day and seven days in the week – that's 168 hours at your disposal. Let's say, for simplicity's sake, that you have the luxury of sleeping or resting for ten hours each night. That leaves ninety-eight hours for work, family life, socialising, leisure – and exercise.

Traditionally, people think of exercise in terms of getting in three hour-long 'sessions' per week, whether at the gym, an aerobics class, a game of badminton or a walk. That's using just three waking hours out of a total of ninety-eight, which still leaves ninety-five hours of potentially active time that you aren't making the most of.

Two things are wrong with this model of behaviour:

1. The timings: can you *realistically* expect a *radical* change in health (or body shape or fitness) in just three hours out of a possible ninety-eight per week?

2. Manageability: how easy is it *realistically* to actually carve out those three hours? Three hours might not sound like a lot – it isn't – but it can be surprisingly difficult to find them when you have to juggle other things like family and work deadlines. Then there's the huge question of motivation. There is a reason why so many gym memberships go unused,

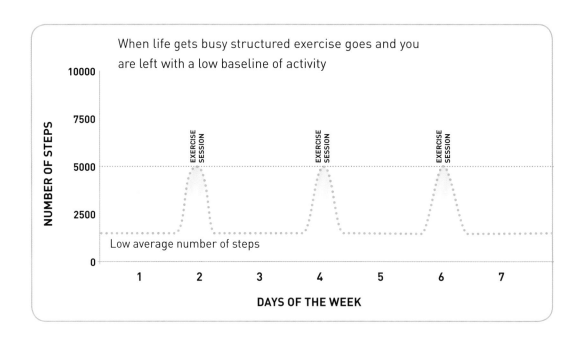

When life gets busy structured exercise goes and you are left with a low baseline of activity

NUMBER OF STEPS

10000
7500
5000
2500
0

EXERCISE SESSION

Low average number of steps

DAYS OF THE WEEK

1   2   3   4   5   6   7

Health Behaviours: the Knock-on Effect

When it comes to your health, how you feel about your behaviour (emotionally) matters – a lot. There is a well-documented knock-on effect between 'health behaviours' such as eating, exercise or other factors, such as whether you smoke or drink a lot of alcohol. In other words, if you feel good about one 'health behaviour' – for instance, your ability to exercise – then you are more likely to behave healthily in other areas of your life. Thinking about exercise in terms of three hour-long sessions (say at the gym, an aerobics class or running) can be quite fraught. And whether or not you manage those three sessions is likely to have a big effect on your other health behaviours.

Now, imagine it's Sunday evening and we're having a chat about how you're planning to exercise over the week ahead. If you know you can get three sessions in, you'll feel really good. This positive feeling is then likely to generate other healthy behaviours. Perhaps you'll cook up a fresh vegetable soup instead of ordering a curry for dinner, or maybe you'll decide not to have that second glass of wine.

If you plan to go to the gym three times, but it does not happen, however, you'll probably feel pretty bad. You might feel frustrated, upset, disappointed – as if you've let yourself down. You might think, 'I can't stick to anything', and this will impact on your other health behaviours: the ice-cream tub will start calling or that extra half bottle of wine, the takeaway or the crisp nibbles or you'll jump in the car to run that errand, rather than walking.

The beauty of Walkactive is that because it is integrated into your lifestyle – it's part of how you walk to work, do the school run, walk the dog, get to the shops – you are not trying to 'stick' to a fixed schedule of structured exercise. You are therefore far less likely to get these negative feelings. With Walkactive, you know that you're aiming to up your steps, but you also know that you can do this. And you know that some weeks are better than others – and that's OK. You don't have that 'boom–bust' mentality. So your health behaviours overall are likely to improve, with the knock-on effect working for you, not against you.

and so many New Year's resolutions have fallen flat by the end of January (and often even sooner!): making time for structured exercise 'sessions' – even three per week – is hard to do. It's easy to skip one, two or three of them, or feel too busy, too bored or too fed up when you don't see results. In short, I believe we're chasing the wrong thing when we 'set aside' time to exercise. We're chasing down those three hours – busting a gut for them – when we should be looking at our lives completely differently. It's not about finding three hours per week. It's about how you navigate those ninety-eight active hours at your disposal.

Walkactive allows you to make the most of every step you take, whatever you're doing, and this is cumulatively far more worthwhile than concentrating all your energy on a gym session three times a week. It gives you an active life – hours and hours of it every week. So by working your body effectively during all those hours – as you do with Walkactive – you're going to catapult your body into a completely different zone. And what's more, by integrating exercise into those hours – again, as you do with Walkactive – then when life gets busy it won't drop off the list.

TROUBLESHOOTING

'My health hasn't been great so I'm unfit – I feel daunted that I have to do so much.'
I fully appreciate that if your starting point is total inactivity – zero steps – then 5000 might seem like a huge task. But it is OK – in fact, it's advisable – to build up gradually. So while 5000 steps and 30 minutes' activity is your target, if you are starting from a very low point, you can still get huge benefits while you are working towards these goals. Again, it's all in the consistency of your efforts. And if your starting point is zero, then in many ways you're lucky: you have the biggest gains to make, and you'll feel better really quickly. A little effort can go a *very* long way. (See pages 83–5 for tips on building up your steps, and page 82 for why as little as five minutes can make a huge difference to your daily step count.) Also see Stan's case study on page 102.

'I've had abdominal surgery and I'm finding it hard to locate and use my abdominal muscles.' Abdominal surgery may make it harder to find hip stability and master the hip lift, and also to feel much at all when you start to do your Abdominal Js. You may also feel some discomfort in your shins; this is because you aren't as good at using those core muscles which will shift your centre of gravity away from your lower legs. My advice is to press on with your Abdominal J exercises even though you may not feel any response at first: just by concentrating on this area, and visualising it, pulling in and up to trace that J, you will be establishing a connection between your abdominal muscles (they are still in there) and your brain. In time, those muscles will respond. To speed the process, try the following:

- Do a set of Abdominal Js every day, while standing up. Put the palm of your hand low down over the abdominal area – towards your pubic bone, so you are touching the area where you want the muscles to respond. Repeat this five to ten times daily. Don't rush it – try to stay focused.
- Before each walk, perform three to five Abdominal Js. This will wake up the correct area, even before you've taken a step.

• Work on posture. If you spend most of your day sitting down, then try to do some Abdominal Js before you start any Walkactive walk. This will help your posture so that you do not sit down in your hips – having your weight low in your hips, rather than pulled upwards (the hip lift) will put more pressure on your abdominal area.

MAKING WALKACTIVE WORK FOR COMMON HEALTH PROBLEMS

While Walkactive is a fabulous way to protect your health and prevent future problems, it can also be wonderful for tackling existing health issues. As stated earlier, it is always essential to talk to your doctor before starting any exercise routine, so do discuss Walkactive with your GP or specialist first. Then, once you have the OK from them and can start Walkactive, you may see huge improvements in your health, vitality, symptoms and energy levels.

Walkactive for heart conditions

At first, your priority is going to be technique not pace. Take time perfecting your posture pace and enjoy the fluidity of movement without applying your accelerators. But as your stamina, technique and confidence improve, you can gradually increase the length of your walks. Begin to apply your accelerators so that your pace increases and your heart rate begins to speed up. The key is to increase the length and number of your walks as well as your pace very gradually – maybe over some weeks.

Walkactive for type-2 diabetes

A study published in 2010 in the *American Journal of Nursing* found that although all exercise is beneficial for people with type-2 diabetes, there are added advantages to be gained from walking after dinner (rather than before). The study looked at the effects of twenty-minute walks both before and after dinner and found that when people walked after dinner their blood-sugar levels lowered more than they did with a before-dinner walk. Another study found that a two-hour walk lowered blood sugar 2.3 times more than a one-hour walk. So in other words, walk as much as you can – and after dinner!

Walkactive for high cholesterol

Long-term studies into exercise and cholesterol levels suggest that the amount of exercise you do matters more than the intensity when it comes to lowering levels of 'bad' (LDL) cholesterol. This is really positive news if you aren't a 'natural' exerciser – it means you don't have to thrash it out for miles at a constant OWP to

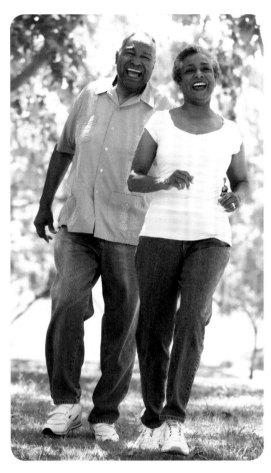

and have found no evidence to suggest that moderate exercise, such as walking, harms the joints. In fact, there is actually significant evidence to show that walking is good for the joints, muscles and bones. Power walking, which increases pressure on the joints, can aggravate joint pain. But with Walkactive, the focus is on the correct joint alignment which could, in fact, reduce symptoms, but should certainly not make them worse.

Walkactive for fatigue

If you are battling with a health issue – or recovering from illness, surgery, treatment or other ailments – you may find that your energy levels are very low. The thought of trying to get out and walk 5000 steps per day might seem impossible right now, but I want you to know that it isn't. You may just have to take it very slowly, and build up a very small number of steps at a time. As you do this, your fitness and energy levels will slowly increase too. This takes patience and determination – but be gentle on yourself and systematically, slowly build up your steps – even if it's over a period of weeks. If you are starting from a very low point, you will see big health gains from doing fewer than 5000 steps at first. The main thing is to try to get out there every day. Even for a short while. You can do this – it *will* help you.

make a difference. The evidence is that to make an impact on cholesterol levels you need to try and walk between 9 and 12 miles (14.5–19.3km) per week. Your daily 5000 Walkactive steps add up to approximately 2 miles (3.2km), so this really is achievable – but you need to do it consistently, every day.

Walkactive for arthritis

Researchers have spent a lot of time looking into the links between exercise and arthritis

'I am forty-five and was diagnosed with painful and debilitating arthritis in my twenties. I have had countless treatments, medications and even recent spinal surgery. I have tried cycling, swimming, Pilates, yoga and aqua aerobics to keep myself mobile, and the pain under control, but the only exercise that I've ever found really good is walking. I walked a lot – even doing half-marathons – and I thought my walking technique was good. I was fast, I had stamina and it kept the arthritis at bay. But nothing can compare to the benefits I have experienced since meeting up with Joanna and starting Walkactive. I feel more mobile and energised, with less pain in my joints because Walkactive has taught me to be more aware of my postural alignment.

'From "open ankles" to "dangly earrings", with the addition of a tray of glasses on the hips (it really does make sense), I now feel taller and more natural and elegant as I walk. It's a long way from the stressed posture of a power walker or race walker. Indeed, with Walkactive you notice that you are no longer pounding the pavement at all: your footfall is lighter and you feel as though you are just skimming the surface. Less pounding means less impact on the joints, knees, hips, lower back and shoulders – and mine all now feel better. I can safely say that Walkactive is the best exercise I have found after twenty-six years of suffering from arthritis.'

SARAH, 45, ATTENDED A WALKACTIVE SPA BREAK

YOU *ARE* WORTH IT

By choosing to do Walkactive for your health you've given yourself a valuable, amazing gift. Walkactive is going to work wonders for your health and well-being – now and for your future. You may already have an illness to cope with, you may be in pain or have mobility issues, or there may be a history of cancer or cardiovascular disease in your family that you are keen to prevent in yourself. Or maybe you just want to feel like a million dollars. Whatever your health objectives, Walkactive is going to help you. All you have to do is follow my programme – get out there every day – and I promise you will see results. You will discover new energy and verve – everything you need to live your best, healthiest life. Now that's surely worth a few extra steps in your day!

CHAPTER SIX

WALKACTIVE FOR FITNESS

'What I'm most surprised about is that I'm finding Walkactive a more effective workout than boot camp. I'm gobsmacked!'

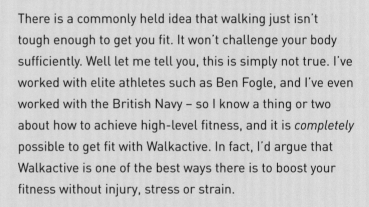

There is a commonly held idea that walking just isn't tough enough to get you fit. It won't challenge your body sufficiently. Well let me tell you, this is simply not true. I've worked with elite athletes such as Ben Fogle, and I've even worked with the British Navy – so I know a thing or two about how to achieve high-level fitness, and it is *completely* possible to get fit with Walkactive. In fact, I'd argue that Walkactive is one of the best ways there is to boost your fitness without injury, stress or strain.

The beauty of getting fit with Walkactive is that you don't just improve your fitness, you improve your technique – and so, as a by-product, your posture and functional health (balance, mobility) improve too. You don't just feel fitter, you feel stronger, tauter and leaner. And you don't risk injury; you guard yourself against it – because with Walkactive, you work *with* your body, not against it. And this just isn't the case with many vigorous fitness training approaches – in fact, with most intensive fitness methods your risk of injury increases along with the intensity of your workout.

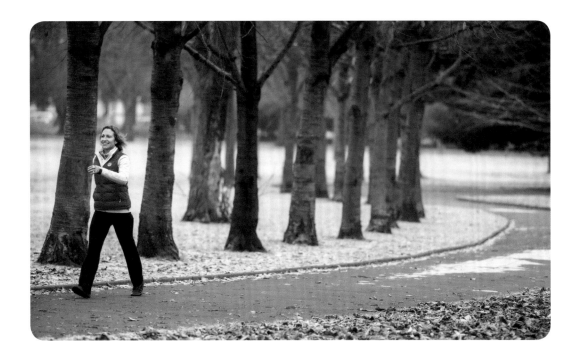

So whether your aim is to become super-fit, to improve your performance in your chosen sport or simply to run for a bus without feeling like you're going to die, Walkactive is going to get you there. Let me show you how.

YOUR WALKACTIVE FOR FITNESS PLAN

First, put on your pedometer! Now here's what you're going to do:

• Walk at least 5000 steps every day using your Walkactive technique and aiming to take at least 115 steps per minute.

• Add three Pace Walks every single week. These can be as short as five minutes if you are starting out (though in total the sessions will be twelve- to fifteen-minutes long as you'll need to do your warm-up and cool-down on either side – see page 120). The key is to get out there walking at your Optimum Walking Pace (OWP) three times per week – that's the fastest possible pace using your perfect technique.

• Follow the twelve-week plan at the end of this chapter. This is because you need a structure – it is vital to keeping you going, progressing and feeling you are working towards something. So stick to the structure!

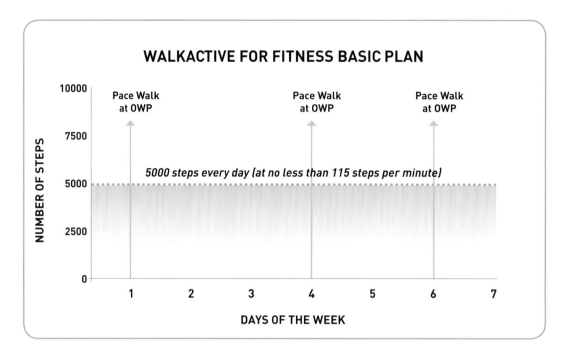

WALKACTIVE FOR FITNESS BASIC PLAN

5000 steps every day (at no less than 115 steps per minute)

Pace Walk at OWP

NUMBER OF STEPS

DAYS OF THE WEEK

FITNESS PACE: THE NEED FOR SPEED

It's worth reminding yourself now about how to switch on and use your accelerators. You aren't just going to walk faster and faster to get fit – you are going to stay true to the technique. This is absolutely crucial because Walkactive brings added value. It isn't just about burning energy. It's about optimising the way your body moves. And this will get you fitter, faster.

You are going to use your toes to propel you forward; focus on your hip lift, so that your legs can extend fully backward, using your bottom muscles powerfully; and you're going to use your arms, so that your torso rotates as you walk. Your pace will increase as you do this, but you will look as if you are gliding over the ground.

Key Technique Points for Fitness Pace

1. **Bow and arrow** (see page 51) – you want to lengthen and pre-stretch your muscles to gain as much power as possible.

2. **Open ankle** (see page 32) – it really is vital for pace!

3. **Arms** – your torso needs to rotate with every step to gain power and speed (see page 55).

Expect effort!

To get fitter your body needs to be pushed beyond its comfort zone. And when you push your body it has to adapt to overcome the stresses you are putting on it. These adaptations are happening at a microscopic cellular level throughout your body as you challenge it (see box below) – and once they've taken place you experience the feeling of 'fitness': that sense of energy and power that you love, whereby you are not out of breath as you run up the stairs, and have more huff and puff for your everyday activities. But to get to this point you have to endure a certain amount of physical discomfort.

All of these changes happen as you get fitter, but they don't all happen at once, nor do they happen steadily. This is why, to increase your fitness you need to find different ways to challenge your body. You need to keep pushing it, so that it keeps adapting.

Your Body's Fitness Adaptations

As you push your body and it starts to adapt in order to cope with the demands placed upon it, the following will take place:

- **Your body will produce more blood capillaries in the lining of the lungs.** These give the lungs a greater surface area, helping more oxygen to pass through from your lungs into your bloodstream, where it is rushed to the working muscles for more energy.

- **More enzymes will be released.** These are important chemical catalysts which, among other things, help your body to turn oxygen and carbohydrates into energy.

- **More mitochondria will be produced.** These are the 'factory assembly plants' in your cells where energy is made.

- **A greater network of blood capillaries is formed throughout the body.** This carries the nutrient-rich blood that will bring energy to those working muscles (it will also help your body to remove waste products).

- **Your heart is strengthened.** In particular, this affects the left side, so that it can expel more blood with each beat. This, in turn, reduces the pressure on your heart (it is beating faster because of the work you are doing). The heart tissue itself will also grow more capillaries so that it can supply itself with more energy and nutrients.

HOW FIT ARE YOU NOW?

When you start out on this Walkactive fitness challenge, it's important to establish how fit you are now. This gives you a way to track your progress. There are two ways to do this – one simple, the other more sophisticated. I've given you both below, so you have a choice, but I always opt for the simple version ('Simple timed fitness test') with my clients as it's easier to use. If, however, you want to see how you rate in terms of your age too, then the 'One-mile walk test' is a great measure.

Simple timed fitness test

- Map out a set distance – about 1km is ideal, though if you are a complete novice to walking and exercise 0.5km is fine too.
- Walk this distance *as fast as you can,* recording the time it takes you, and rate how difficult it felt on a scale of one to ten (see the Effort Scale opposite).
- Do this on Day 1 and every month or so – it's a good way to see how you are progressing. Walk the exact same route and note the improvement!

You could also record your heart rate with a heart-rate monitor if you have one, but if you want to do this make sure you get readings for sixty seconds before you start the timed distance walk, sixty seconds after you finish it, and then, after recovering for a minute, another sixty seconds. Record your heart rate at each of these points. Also record the time it took and how it felt.

Remember: walk the distance *as fast as possible* to get a true indication of your fitness level.

One-mile walk test

This test was developed by researchers as a way to establish aerobic fitness, which is a good indicator of overall fitness.
You will need:

- a stopwatch or watch that indicates seconds
- a flat, measured route that is 1 mile (1.6km) long without hills, roads to cross or traffic lights; walking round the block is fine.

Here's how you do the test:

1. Do a four- to five-minute warm-up using your Walkactive technique.
2. Note your start time. Now, walk the mile as fast as you can (but at a steady pace). You may not have mastered your OWP the first time you do this; it increases the better you get at Walkactive.
3. At the end of the mile note your time in minutes and seconds.

Test ratings
Women

Age	20-29	30-39	40-49	50-59	60-69	70+
Excellent	< 13:12	< 13:42	< 14:12	< 14:42	< 15:06	< 18:18
Good	13:12-14:06	13:42-14:36	14:12-15:06	14:42-15:36	15:06-16:18	18:18-20:00
Average	14:07-15:06	14:37-15:36	15:07-16:06	15:37-17:00	16:19-17:30	20:01-21:48
Fair	15:07-16:30	15:37-17:00	16:07-17:30	17:01-18:06	17:31-19:12	21:49-24:06
Poor	>16:30	>17:00	>17:30	>18:06	>19:12	>24:06

Men

Age	20-29	30-39	40-49	50-59	60-69	70+
Excellent	< 11:54	< 12:24	< 12:54	< 13:24	< 14:06	< 15:06
Good	11:54-13:00	12:24-13:30	12:54-14:00	13:24-14:24	14:06-15:12	15:06-15:48
Average	13:01-13:42	13:31-14:12	14:01-14:42	14:25-15:12	15:13-16:18	15:49-18:48
Fair	13:43-14:30	14:13-15:00	14:43-15:30	15:13-16:30	16:19-17:18	18:49-20:18
Poor	>14:30	>15:00	>15:30	>16:30	>17:18	>20:18

Key: < less than; > more than. Note: all times are in minutes and seconds.

Effort Scale

You can also monitor your heart rate or how much effort you feel the test called for on a scale of one to ten, where:

0	no effort at all
0.5	almost no effort
1	very little effort
2	a little more effort, but still very easy to maintain
3	moderate effort (this is equivalent to your posture pace – while you may not feel out of breath, you'll be aware that you are using your body effectively)
4	a bit more effort (your breathing is faster; you are feeling slightly warmer)
5	strong effort (this is around the start of your OWP range)
6/7	stronger effort (you are working hard, breathing fast)
7/8	even stronger (this is the top end of your OWP - you're walking as fast as you can without compromising your technique, your breathing is fast, your limbs feel as if they are working almost as hard as they can)
9/10	maximum effort (you are walking as fast as you can, but your movement is snatched, tense and stiff, your postural alignment is compromised, you are very out of breath – you won't be able to maintain your technique)

You may feel disappointed by your fitness level, or you may be surprised that you are fitter than you'd thought. It doesn't matter – this is just your starting point. You are going to get fitter from hereon in, whatever your level is now. You just need to record where you are so you can track your progress.

Take a little notebook with you (or use your Smartphone or other electronic device) and make sure you note down your times and effort levels. You can then test yourself again after four weeks, and you'll see the progress you've made.

Measuring OWP steps per minute

As you start the Fitness Plan it is a good idea to measure your steps per minute when you are using your OWP (see page 62 for full details). This is another way to track your progress. This is what you do:

- Warm up for five to eight minutes, using your Walkactive technique.
- Do a break-point drill (see page 62) to establish your true OWP.
- Walk at your OWP for one to three minutes. You're not measuring anything here – you just want to be confident that this really is the right pace for you. Then stop.

- Now set your pedometer to zero. You're going to record your steps per minute.
- Walk for sixty seconds at your OWP. The number showing on your pedometer when you have done this is your OWP steps per minute.

I want you to record your OWP steps per minute at the start of your Fitness Plan, then after four weeks and then again after eight weeks. You should see an interesting pattern: your steps per minute will probably increase for about a month as you get fitter. But then, as your technique improves, your steps per minute will start to decrease. This is because your strides will lengthen. If you see this happening, it's great news! When your Walkactive technique increases the length of your strides, your body is working harder – and so it's getting fitter. It's no good just forcing yourself to take longer strides though; if you do this, you'll use the wrong muscles. The longer strides have to evolve as you master the technique.

FITNESS-BOOSTING WALKS

To increase the intensity and speed of your Pace Walks I want you to include some fitness-boosting sessions in your Fitness Plan. These will focus on speed, slopes and timing. They will challenge and push your

CASE STUDY: NICOLA – FORCED TO STOP RUNNING

Nicola was always super-fit. Her first degree was in dance and choreography, she did Ashtanga yoga on and off for years, started running in her twenties – long distances, including marathons – and swam competitively. However, two years ago, serious back problems forced her to give up running just weeks away from the London Marathon. She was utterly devastated. She couldn't run, and her back problems meant that she also had pain and weakness in one leg and one arm, so her swimming style was ruined too. 'I basically lay on the floor for two months and wept. My kids were like, "Oh yeah, Mum's crying again." I couldn't run and swimming felt horrible and slow, hard and so uncompetitive. I just couldn't come to terms with performing at a lower ability.'

Nicola knew that she needed to find an activity that she could do outdoors and which was challenging, but also low-impact and core-strengthening (the only way to prevent the pain in her leg and lower back). Luckily, she discovered Walkactive! 'It makes complete sense to me and to my body,' she says. 'It is an incredible workout. It works on my body from the inside out – my waist has lengthened and shrunk, my stomach has flattened and my buttocks feel rock hard. I think I may have even shaved a few centimetres off my thighs – it's unbelievable. I feel powerful and strong now. One of the best things is that Walkactive is transferable to all areas of my life. I use my Abdomimal Js all the time: when walking, or at the computer, or around the house. I use the Walkactive technique while doing the Hoovering or cooking or teaching. It's really a state of being: a lifestyle. One of the brilliant things about Walkactive is that everyone can do it, whatever their fitness level. But the most surprising thing to me was how, as a very fit person, I still feel so physically stretched by Walkactive.'

'I feel powerful and strong now. One of the best things is that Walkactive is transferable to all areas of my life. I use my Abdomimal Js all the time: when walking, or at the computer, or around the house.'

body, increasing your fitness levels, while maintaining your technique. (See the plan on page 132 for when to incorporate them.)

One route – three ways

This is a one-off addition to your Pace Walks and your 5000 daily steps. It takes about an hour. I want you to do this in phase one of your Fitness Plan – and then again the following month. After this, you can continue to do 'One route – three ways' monthly to check your progress.

'One route – three ways' is great for increasing your pace, but it also teaches you something about your Walkactive technique. It is a way to monitor your pace and stride length as you get fitter. You may find that your fastest time actually comes when you are aiming to use fewer steps: as your stride lengthens, you'll be covering more ground per step; you are also pre-lengthening your muscles (remember the bow and arrow, see page 51) and this propels you forward. This lengthened stride uses more energy – it challenges your muscles and, in so doing, increases your fitness.

How to do it

You'll need your pedometer and a route that takes you twenty minutes to walk at a normal, posture pace. It can be a loop of your park, an out/back route to your home

or several trips round the block. It just needs to be a distance that you can repeat. You are going to walk this route three times. Take your pedometer and a little notebook or a Smartphone with you. After each walk, note down your time and step count. Then reset your pedometer.

I want you to focus on a different element of the Walkactive technique during each of the three route walks:

- **Walk 1: pace** Walk your route as fast as you can (obviously, it will now take you less than twenty minutes when you are walking at your OWP rather than posture pace). Record your time
- **Walk 2: technique** Technique is always crucial, but here your focus is on technique more than ever, without worrying too much about pace. Record your time.
- **Walk 3: stride length** Walk your route using fewer steps (lengthen your stride). Record your time.

 Warm up and cool down

- *Start with five minutes practising your technique, to warm up.*
- *After each route, do five Abdominal Js – this should take no longer than sixty seconds.*
- *Finish the last walk with a two- to four-minute cool-down at your posture pace.*

When you repeat this session after a month, you'll notice quite a difference to your steps and pace. But remember, your best speed is not 'best' if your body is tense and your technique is snatched. You'll be compromising your posture and joint alignment and will miss out on the maximum potential shape-change or fitness benefits. Stay true to the technique!

Slopes-and-stride drill

I love slopes. Yes, they do make you work harder, but they are a great way to perfect your Walkactive technique – particularly its muscle-lengthening effect – while simultaneously providing a fantastic cardiovascular workout. You can include this drill in your Pace Walks to give yourself a fitness boost.

How to do it

You'll need to find a gradual slope – one where you appreciate it is an incline, but it is not so steep that you have to lean from the hip to get up the hill. Choose a distance of about 50–75 metres up the slope. You are going to be walking up and down this one stretch. Now, here's what you do (also see 'Walkactive on Slopes', on page 122):

- Do a five-minute warm-up before you start: practise your open-ankle position and add your Abdominal Js. Try to really feel the bow-and-arrow effect – your muscles lengthening with every stride.
- Now start walking up the slope. Focus on your stride length, your open ankle and hip lift. Don't worry about speed. At the top, turn around and walk down again, making sure you are lifting out of the hips.
- Turn around and repeat. This time count the number of steps you take to reach the top. (I find it easier to just count every right stride!) At the top, turn around and walk down again. No need to count this time – just focus on lengthening your stride.

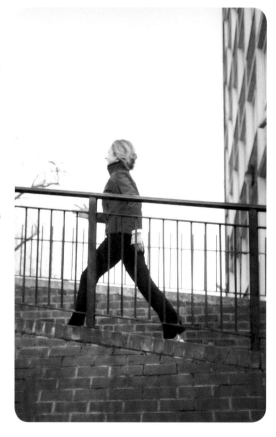

Walkactive on Slopes

People often ask me if you can really still do the technique when you're walking uphill. Of course you can! But you will need to focus on slightly different body parts. If you do this as you walk up slopes you will give yourself a really challenging cardiovascular workout and your technique will come on in leaps and bounds.

On hills, the important thing to remember – as always – is: never compromise your technique. The four basic elements of the Walkactive technique still apply on slopes (your feet, hips, neck and shoulders and arms), but your focus should shift slightly from your feet to your hips. When you are walking on a flat pavement, your feet are most definitely the most important part of the technique. But as you start to walk up a slope, it becomes even more important to get the hip lift right.

Walking up the slope

• Lead from the open ankle, peeling your foot off the floor. Don't let your hips do all the work.

• Focus on drawing up and out of your hips. Imagine you have a pair of wings on your back and you're gliding up the hill, rather than dragging yourself up by leaning over at your hip crease.

• Try to keep length in your torso – make as much space as you can between your pubic bone and your breast bone; don't hunch or lean over as you walk. This is a lengthening, stretching in your torso – you aren't bending over at the hips to haul yourself up the hill. That belly button is lifted.

• On a steeper hill your stride may have to get a little shorter, but keep pulling up and out of your hips, lifting that belly button up – this will safeguard your knees and keep you in the correct postural alignment. Don't hunch!

Walking down the slope

• Don't lean back and sink into your hips – this will put greater pressure on your lower back.

• When we walk downhill we tend to shorten our stride and sit down into the hips. This puts pressure on both hips and knees. I want you to focus on lifting up and out of the hips, keeping your stride longer as you come down. So as you walk downhill, imagine you have a piece of string tied around your big toe. This string is pulling you gently down the slope. Picturing this in your mind will help you to lengthen your stride.

• Keep your upper body lifted and use your Abdominal Js – this will allow your legs to move freely.

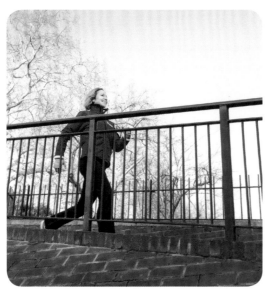

- Repeat twice more: each time your target is to take at least two strides off your previous total. So you're walking the same distance up that slope, but you're going to do it in fewer steps. To do this, you'll have to lift up from your hips, peel through your whole foot, keeping an open ankle, and make sure your upper body stays relaxed.

This is simple, yet fabulous. The emphasis is on lengthening your stride and not racing up the slope as fast as possible, but you'll find it is an amazing cardiovascular workout – your breathing and heart rate will increase, and you'll get warmer. Your muscle fibres are working much harder when they are in this extended position (that's the longer, more effective strides). Try it – it will pay dividends for your fitness and your technique.

'I was roped into Walkactive by my wife – she basically wanted company. I did it to be nice. I consider myself pretty fit – I was running a few miles three times a week, and had a game of squash with my brother at least once. But to be honest, my knees were playing up, I'd had disc problems, and I knew running wasn't going to be sustainable for me in the long term. Still, it never occurred to me for a moment that I could improve my fitness just by walking. I was astonished at how hard my body was able to work at Walkactive without the pain I'd usually have from running. In just two to three weeks I was feeling the difference in my energy levels – and my torso slimmed down a bit too. I decided to stop running, and see what happened. I thought I'd see some kind of decrease in fitness, but my fitness has continued to improve and my pace too – and I'm thrashing my brother at squash.'

DAVE, 54, WALKACTIVE CLUB MEMBER

Interval walks

Interval walks vary the speed and intensity at which your body works. This not only increases the number of calories you'll burn, but is also amazingly good for your heart: interval training can double and even triple the heart-protecting benefits you get from moderate-intensity exercise sessions (even when you exercise for less time).

Short bursts of high-intensity walking can also:

- make your heart work harder and pump more blood with each beat, which strengthens your entire cardiovascular system, increasing your fitness and promoting heart health
- stimulate your muscles to develop more mitochondria (the energy-producing 'factories' within your cells that use sugar and fat for fuel); the more of these you have, the better your muscles become at using carbohydrates (you burn more calories!) and this process also improves your body's blood-sugar balance
- potentially reduce your blood pressure – when you do interval work, your artery walls produce nitric oxide, and this helps them to dilate so that blood flows more easily through them.

How to do it

The best way to make sure you are really working hard enough on your high-intensity bursts is to use the effort scale on page 117 (where one is equal to sitting on the sofa watching TV, while ten is all out, as fast as you can go – although obviously, I'm not asking you to do this, as your technique would be shot to pieces at that effort level). To reach the higher-intensity end of your scale, try adding inclines, as well as perfecting your bow-and-arrow lengthened muscles (this comes as you really master the technique).

Interval Walking – Suggested Workout

This is another way to add interest to your Pace Walks. Over a six-week period:

Weeks 1–3: alternate between one minute at effort level 7–8 and one minute at 5–6. Do this nine times.

Weeks 4–6: alternate between two minutes at effort level 7–8 and one minute at 5–6. Do this seven times.

Suggested Pattern for Bursts of High-/Moderate-intensity Walking

Activity	Time	Effort level
Warm-up	5 minutes	4–5
Intervals	18 minutes minimum	Alternate bursts of high- and moderate-intensity walking (see suggested pattern above)
Cool-down	3 minutes	4–5

'4 x 10' session

I love this session and my clients seem to love it too! Bursts of more intense speed help you to work on your OWP, so really stretching yourself. They increase your stamina, challenge your body and therefore improve your fitness.

You may find that you don't like the idea of having to do the route four times, but as your technique improves, your times will speed up. This is highly rewarding and motivating. It's amazing to see your progress in actual concrete numbers. It will make you realise one important thing: you really can do this!

How to do it

You need to find a route that will take you anywhere between five and ten minutes to walk at posture pace. If it's less than five, you'll start to miss the point of the drill and you won't get the same cardiovascular benefits; more than ten, and the session in total takes longer than fifty minutes – that's a big ask in our time-pressed lives, and you may have guessed that I'm a big fan of optimising your efforts!

Now, here's what you do:

• Start with a five-minute technique warm-up.

• Next, walk the route at your OWP and record your time.
• Take forty-five seconds to recover – ideally, doing your standing Abdominal Js as you do so.
• Repeat the route three more times, aiming to reduce the time taken for each one.
• Finish with a two- to four-minute cool-down at your posture pace.

'4 x 10': Great for Groups!

This is an excellent session to do on your own, but I find it especially effective when I'm working with a group or team. If you're training for a charity distance walk, you might want to involve your friends, or if you are doing Walkactive as a group for motivation and encouragement, then do this session together. Simply record the time of the first person to reach the distance and the last person: this gives you a time range – your fastest and slowest time. Your aim is to reduce this time range. So say your fastest group member did the route in 10.10 seconds and your slowest came in at 11.15 seconds, on your second attempt you want your fastest group member to come in at less than 10.10 seconds and your last person to cross the 'finish line' in less than 11.15 seconds. This way everyone stays motivated and you have to work as a team.

WALK TIME TRIALS

I'm a big fan of completing a timed longer-distance route once a month: it's a fabulous way to challenge yourself and monitor your progress. It is great to have your monthly Walk Time Trial pencilled in your diary, so that even if life gets busy you make it happen. This way, you won't lose sight of your fitness goals. Walk Time Trials are also the perfect way to complement your training if you are doing a charity distance walk.

Seven-kilometre Walk Time Trials are a regular feature of the Walkactive events I run with my team; 7km may sound like a long way, but there are good reasons for this:

- While 5km might seem quite manageable and 10km a bit of a trek, 7km is somewhere in between – a distance at which you'll be pushed, but it won't take you for ever to complete. So you can do it, and still be home in time to put the Sunday roast in the oven – you'll feel so virtuous!
- Walking 7km at your OWP is a fabulous training stimulus: you are pushing yourself all the time, as you're not allowed to stop or ease off. This is a performance: there is a 'ready steady go', then you're walking until you reach the chequered flag! This is mental and physical training – endurance and speed.

Walkactive Walk Time Trials

These are group events, held in different parts of the country to which everyone is welcome. We get plenty of people who are completely new to Walkactive, but we also get regulars who need a fitness boost or who want feedback on their technique from me or one of my Walkactive trainers.

The fastest time we have ever had for completing one of our 7km routes is just under forty-four minutes and we generally get everyone back within ninety. It is a deeply rewarding, social and motivating event because you also get to see the changes in other people as their Walkactive journeys evolve.

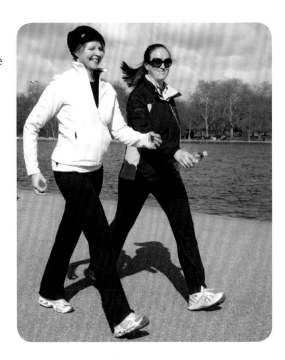

'I signed up for La Manga as soon as I read a Guardian *article about it. I booked ten months ahead! In the interim I began to swim and run more, and did a military-style boot camp. I'm quite fit and before I went to La Manga I was a bit worried Walkactive wouldn't be hard enough for me. How wrong I was. I was pushed within an inch of my life. When the La Manga course finished I was thinking, 'I'll use this technique when I'm walking, but I'll go back to boot camp for the adrenaline rush.' But then I did a boot-camp class and it was really irritating. What I was taught there was completely at odds with Walkactive; I realised I'd get a cardiovascular workout, but that was about it. I wasn't using my body fully at all. I knew then that I was properly converted to the benefits of the Walkactive technique. What I'm most surprised about, however, is that I'm finding Walkactive a more effective workout than boot camp. I'm gobsmacked!'*

NICOLA, 42, ATTENDED WALKACTIVE
TRAINING CAMP

ADVICE TO RUNNERS AND REGULARS

If you are a runner or a committed walker, you will probably have a natural stride – a rhythm of your own – and you'll automatically switch into that as you walk. This is great in some ways because it means you can comfortably get going – you switch on autopilot and you're off.

However, the downside of this natural rhythm is that you may find it hard to adjust to the Walkactive lengthened stride. If your stride stays short, you will miss out on many of the cardiovascular and shape-changing benefits of Walkactive. You are also probably already very tight in your hip flexors and this will keep your stride shorter too. And if you are covering distance quickly by taking shorter, more frequent steps, you are basically power walking: and this is a big no-no.

So I really want you to concentrate on the technique so that your stride lengthens. It may feel as if you're slowing down at first, but that doesn't matter. What matters is that you stretch and lengthen those muscles, staying true to the technique – and take longer strides. Remember: you're aiming to speed up using fewer steps, not more of them.

WALKACTIVE ADVANCED TECHNIQUE

If you feel that you've really mastered your Walkactive basic technique – that is, you're totally confident, it feels smooth and natural and you are getting on well with your three weekly Pace Walks – then you could be ready for something more advanced.

Walkactive Advanced Technique will improve your fitness, shape, posture and joints further still and bring you even more health benefits. So when you're ready, give it a try.

There are three parts to the Advanced Technique:

1. Foot absorption The longer you keep your foot on the ground, the more it will propel

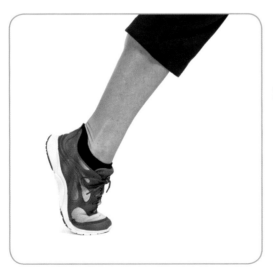

Foot Absorption: the Science

Physiologically, what's happening here is quite mind-blowing: the arch of your foot has receptors on it which, when stimulated, encourage greater muscle contraction. Basically, they make the muscles on the backs of your legs and your bottom (your hamstrings and glutes) work harder. So the more your feet 'absorb' the ground, the more you'll be stimulating the correct muscles. If you rush your feet you won't actually reach your OWP, but if you concentrate on foot absorption, you'll increase your pace and your glide. Your body will be working that much harder.

you forward. This is called foot absorption – it's as if your foot is absorbing the ground. Keeping your foot down to move faster probably sounds wrong, but trust me: you'll get more power and pace this way. Try it and see: slow down your stride and really make your foot absorb the ground, peeling it slowly off the ground.

2. Hip angle Your stride will be getting longer and your hips will be opening more. In the perfect Walkactive stride your front leg will be at the same angle as your back leg (see photograph above right), with your upper body symmetrically balanced in the middle. To start with, you may find your hip flexors are tight: this will mean you can't open at the hips as

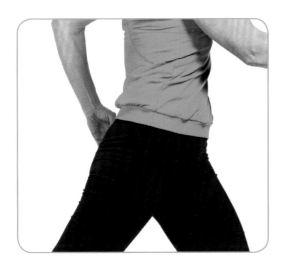

well and so your leg will not stretch back as far as you move. But as you perfect the technique, your hips will open up, allowing for this symmetrical stride.

3. Spine rotation As you relax through your neck and shoulders, you'll become more aware of the relationship between your hip lift and your shoulders and neck – remember that physical oxymoron? You're lifting up your hips, but relaxing the shoulders. As you get better at this, your shoulders will start to open up at the front. And then, as you swing your arms, the movement will come from all the way across your shoulders rather than just from the shoulder joint. This means that not only are you whittling your waist more effectively, you are also becoming more aerodynamic. Your body isn't completely facing the direction that

you're moving in as you walk forward; it is slicing the air, one shoulder at a time. You're therefore exposing less of your body to wind resistance. Result: your pace increases. If this is hard to visualise, think about a freestyle (crawl) swimmer: their torso rotates in the water with each stroke, making them travel forward faster. If your spine is doing this – rotating as in the photograph below – it is allowing you to walk faster. The faster pace will use more energy and boost your cardiovascular fitness – and, of course, there will be a huge toning bonus all over your body.

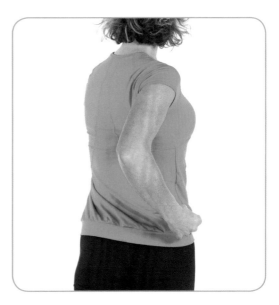

A word of warning: don't rush to Advanced Technique

Do be wary with the Advanced Technique. There is no point rushing into it. Walkactive is all about the process, and you can get amazing benefits as you go along. You don't have to leap to the most advanced parts of the technique to see changes to your fitness. If you try to twist your spine or get a longer stride without putting the whole Walkactive process together properly first, you'll be switching on the wrong muscles, using them in the wrong way and in the wrong sequence. You will just be replacing one 'walking wrong' method with another and you won't see the radical results.

So be patient and enjoy the journey. If you're not doing Walkactive with softness, smoothness and fluidity yet, then you're not ready for the Advanced Technique. Save it for later!

COMMON ROADBLOCKS TO FITNESS

Building fitness is unlikely to be plain sailing. There will always be challenges and setbacks. But you can handle them and keep going – here are the most common ones and how to get past them.

Motivation

It can be hard to keep going with a fitness plan: you might get bored, think it's not working or simply get distracted by life.

That's why I've given you so many sessions to measure your progress. They're not optional add-ons. You really should schedule them in and do them because this way you'll see – in black and white, in numbers no less – that you are making progress. You'll see that your cardiovascular fitness and your body's ability to do the technique are improving, your muscles are lengthening and toning and your alignment is working to push you towards your fitness goals, not away from them.

So keep up the monitoring. A little Walkactive notebook recording all your different times and effort levels will be the perfect motivator, so you can see clearly how you're making amazing progress.

Injury

I talked about this earlier, but it's important to remind yourself of why Walkactive is such a brilliant way to get fit. Nothing will scupper a fitness plan more effectively than an injury – and injuries are very common when you're pushing your body beyond its comfort zone. If you injure yourself, generally you have to stop exercising, or at least take a big step back. This will prevent you from reaching your goals. But with Walkactive, injuries are *extremely* rare. You may get some shin soreness as you master the technique and start to work on your core strength. But we are working with your body's alignment, strengthening it from the inside out and moving it in the way it is designed to move. Injury should simply *not* be an issue with Walkactive. Activities such as yoga, where the focus is on opening up the body, can also be helpful. This will improve the range of motion in your ankles and other joints.

In the unlikely event that you do sprain or strain any part of your body, the best approach is RICE (rest, ice, compression, elevation):

- **R**est: this does not necessarily mean total immobilisation, or weeks on crutches, but it does mean resting your injured body part in the first twenty-four to forty-eight hours post-injury, and going gently and slowly on it afterwards until it is fully healed.
- **I**ce: icing an injury reduces pain by slowing down the transmission of pain signals along the nerves from the injured area to the central nervous system. It can also reduce inflammation.
- **C**ompression: wrapping the injured area firmly in a bandage (or any wrap you have) can greatly reduce the amount of swelling. Swelling is a major factor in prolonged rehabilitation.
- **E**levation: keep the injured body part higher than or equal to the level of your heart. For an ankle sprain, this means

propping your foot up while lying down or sitting. This also reduces swelling.

The treatment undertaken within the first twenty-four hours of an injury can literally cut weeks off your total recovery time, so RICE really matters.

Lack of time

Yes, you are busy. I get it! That's why you need to have a fitness plan and follow it. You need to set times when you know you can go out on your Pace Walks during the week – even if each one is just fifteen minutes long. You also need to schedule in your other sessions. A diary is your best protection against 'lack of time': write down your sessions as you're thinking about the week ahead, and remember, you are building Walkactive into your life – it's how you move around from now on. As you increase your Walkactive pace going about your daily life, you'll notice your fitness increases too. You're working all the time.

Not seeing results

One reason people don't see results when they start a fitness plan is that they don't have a structure – so they let things slip; they kid themselves that they've done enough, or the way they go about it becomes a bit ad-hoc. This is why I want you to have a plan and stick to it.

YOUR TWELVE-WEEK WALKACTIVE FITNESS PLAN

To help you put all this into practice, here is a suggested fitness plan. I've divided it into three four-week phases: it is much easier to follow if it's broken down. Remember, this is in addition to your 5000 steps per day, at 115 steps per minute. If at any time you are finding this too easy or too difficult, simply adjust the length of your Pace Walks accordingly or decrease or lengthen the intensity of your slope work but ensure you do the 5000 steps and four Pace Walks outlined on the basic plan on page 114.

Phase One: lift off

Week one	Pace Session 1: complete fitness test (see page 116) and record results
	Complete a five-minute Pace Walk
	Pace Session 2: complete a ten-minute Pace Walk
	Pace Session 3: complete a five-minute Pace Walk
Week two	Pace Session 1: complete a seven-minute Pace Walk
	Pace Session 2: complete a ten-minute Pace Walk
	Pace Session 3: complete a seven-minute Pace Walk
Week three	Pace Session 1: complete 'One route – three ways' session
	Pace Session 2: complete a ten-minute Pace Walk
	Pace Session 3: complete your first 'Slopes-and-stride' session
Week four	Pace Session 1: complete a Walk Time Trial and record time; aim for a distance of between 3 and 7km. Make a note of your route, so you can repeat it in phases 2 and 3
	Pace Session 2: complete a 'Slopes-and-stride' session
	Pace Session 3: complete a twelve-minute Pace Walk

Phase Two: blasting upward

Week five	Pace Session 1: take it easy this week; it's about consolidating. Complete a twelve-minute Pace Walk
	Pace Session 2: complete a 'Slopes-and-stride' session
	Pace Session 3: complete a twelve-minute Pace Walk

Week six	Pace Session 1: complete 'One route – three ways'
	Pace Session 2: complete fifteen minutes at OWP
	Pace Session 3: complete fifteen minutes at OWP
Week seven	Pace Session 1: complete 'Slopes-and-stride' session, plus five minutes at OWP
	Pace Session 2: complete fifteen minutes at OWP
	Pace Session 3: complete a '4 x 10' session
Week eight	Pace Session 1: complete your Walk Time Trial route and record time
	Pace Session 2: complete '4 x 10' session
	Pace Session 3: complete 'Slopes-and-stride' session, plus five minutes at OWP

Phase Three: reach the clouds

Week nine	Pace Session 1: complete a '4 x 10' session
	Pace Session 2: complete seventeen minutes at OWP
	Pace Session 3: complete 'Slopes-and-stride' session, plus eight minutes at OWP
Week ten	Take it easy this week; it's about consolidation. Repeat all sessions as week nine
Week eleven	Pace Session 1: complete a '4 x 10' session
	Pace Session 2: complete twenty minutes at OWP
	Pace Session 3: complete 'One route – three ways'
Week twelve	Pace Session 1: complete a 'Slopes-and-stride' session, plus twenty minutes at OWP
	Pace Session 2: complete twenty minutes at OWP
	Pace Session 3: complete your Walk Time Trial route and record time

Coping with setbacks

If you miss a week or session, don't panic: just repeat the previous week – think of it as a consolidating week. This is a progressive fitness plan; I'm training you like an athlete. I'm pushing your body safely, so that you get benefits on all levels: posturally, functionally and for your stamina. You'll be amazed at the results, if you follow my plan!

CASE STUDY: KIRSTEN – FITNESS FOR LIFE

At forty-seven, Kirsten was fit and active. A size-ten ex-smoker, she was walking 7–10km every day. When she first heard about Walkactive she was about to embark on a three-day, 150km charity walk through the mountains of Bosnia Herzegovina in extreme heat. She booked a one-to-one session with me just before she set off. 'I crossed the finish line having incorporated what Joanna had taught me into every step along the way,' she says. And as soon as she got back to the UK she signed up for two back-to-back Walkactive courses in Hyde Park in London.

But her life was about to change. A medical check-up showed that one of her heart's arteries was narrowing. 'I was put on drugs including beta blockers and aspirin, most of which gave me side-effects. I couldn't comprehend why this was happening to me. I was fit and young.'

When her cardiologist commented on how fit she was, she told him about her walking – he told her to keep it up because her fitness was what had saved her from needing a stent. 'I can honestly say this doctor's advice – and Walkactive – helped change my life,' she says. 'He showed me my heart on the computer screen. He knew I was fit because there were extra veins surrounding my heart. My walking had created a safety net that I could actually see with my own eyes. A light bulb went on in my head at that moment – I've always known how much better it feels to be fit, but I finally saw the health benefits of being fitter too. The doctor's parting words to me were: "Keep doing what you are doing".'

Kirsten has now been on several Walkactive courses. She's seen her fitness increase even more since she last saw her cardiologist. 'I love the Walkactive classes,' she says. 'I can already see changes in my posture and body; plus, I just feel great. I am hooked!'

Kirsten's story is what Walkactive for fitness is all about. By getting fitter, you not only increase your performance and energy, you improve your health too. You boost your body from the inside out. So if ever you need an extra bit of motivation, think about Kirsten. Imagine your heart getting bigger and stronger inside your chest with every Walkactive session. You can do this. It's not easy, it takes effort, but the benefits are stupendous!

CHAPTER SEVEN

WALKACTIVE FOR INCH LOSS

'I was amazed to find that I'd trimmed nearly 2 inches [5cm] off my waistline – without radically changing my diet! I was thrilled. I was not expecting results so quickly!'

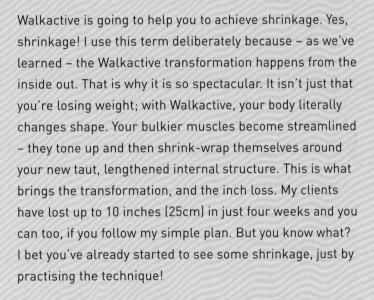

Walkactive is going to help you to achieve shrinkage. Yes, shrinkage! I use this term deliberately because – as we've learned – the Walkactive transformation happens from the inside out. That is why it is so spectacular. It isn't just that you're losing weight; with Walkactive, your body literally changes shape. Your bulkier muscles become streamlined – they tone up and then shrink-wrap themselves around your new taut, lengthened internal structure. This is what brings the transformation, and the inch loss. My clients have lost up to 10 inches (25cm) in just four weeks and you can too, if you follow my simple plan. But you know what? I bet you've already started to see some shrinkage, just by practising the technique!

WEIGHT LOSS OR INCH LOSS?

I want to be clear here: you can lose weight with Walkactive – you just have to read the fabulous success stories here and on my website to know that weight loss is achievable.

Weight is a very emotive subject, but what continually astounds my clients is not the figure they see on the bathroom scales, but the difference they see and feel in their bodies – jeans getting looser, torsos slimming and elongating, bottoms tightening and lifting. This concrete, amazing feeling is far more uplifting than standing every day on a set of scales and hoping to see the numbers shift a bit. If you follow the plan in this chapter, you will see both inch loss and weight loss. I guarantee it. But the greatest difference is going to be where it matters most – in inch loss.

'The thing that has amazed me about Walkactive is how easily it's become part of my life. I've done a million diets in my time, and endless exercise fads – from boxing to karate – and although some worked, I never stuck with them. Each time I'd get fed up and the weight would pile back on. But this is totally different. I've built Walkactive into my daily life – my commute, the school run, my shopping trips. I'm more active than ever before, but I'm not forcing myself and I never count a single calorie. I've gone down from a size sixteen to a size twelve in seven months and I absolutely love how my body feels.'

ROSALYND, 38, WALKACTIVE CLUB MEMBER

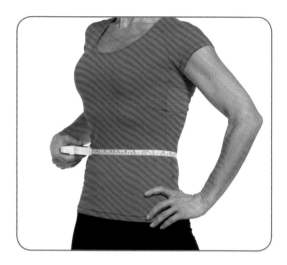

YOUR WALKACTIVE FOR INCH LOSS PLAN

We're going to launch a three-pronged attack, comprised as follows:

- Increased daily steps: you'll need to walk 7500 steps per day – *every* day.
- Pace Walks: complete four *every* week.
- Eating changes: apply my number-one nutritional change – the Carb Curfew (see box opposite) – along with the strategies outlined later in the chapter.

None of this is complicated. Stick to my Walkactive for Inch Loss Plan and you *will* see results. But this means no shortcuts: you can't save up your walks and steps and do mega-binge walking at the weekend. You have to reach those 7500 steps per day, plus Pace Walks. That's what brings results.

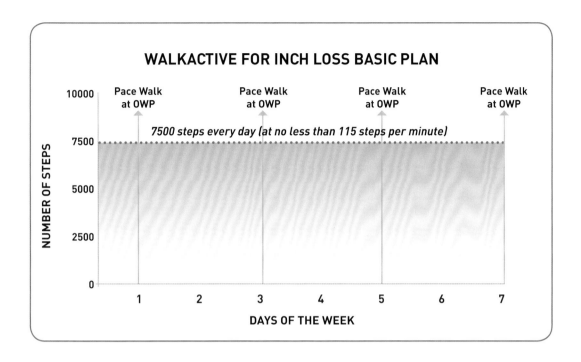

WALKACTIVE FOR INCH LOSS BASIC PLAN

The Carb Curfew

This is my number-one nutritional tool, bringing the greatest changes while leaving you the flexibility to live your life and enjoy your food. And it's simple: you don't eat carbohydrates after 5pm. I'll show you how to make this work a bit later (see page 146).

Take your measurements

Taking your own measurements can be a bit tricky, so you may find it easier to get a friend to help. (Or you can invest in a small, effective self-measuring tape which has a lock valve, so you can easily record each measurement without having to contort yourself to see the tape!) The key here is to measure yourself in exactly the same way each time.

Stand in a neutral position with arms out to the side, level with the shoulders (if someone is measuring you, otherwise – obviously – you'll need your arms!). Ensure the tape is smooth and level at each measuring point.

Women
- Chest: place the tape horizontally around the chest, directly over the nipple line.
- Waist: place the tape around the smallest part of your waist. As a rule that is the midway point between your ribs and pelvis.
- Navel: place the tape directly over the belly button.

- Hips: find the top of your buttocks and take the hip measurement from this point. This may not be your widest part, but it will give you the most consistent measurements as the top of your buttocks won't move!
- Thighs: stand with your feet together. Measure 8 inches (20cm) up from the top of your kneecap and take one circumference measurement around both thighs.

Men

- Chest, hips and thighs: do exactly the same as for women (see above).
- Waist: take two measurements around the belly button – one relaxed and one contracted. First place the tape directly over the belly button when completely relaxed, so the abdominal muscles are extended, but not forced out. Take this measurement. Next, measure the waist contracted by placing the tape horizontally over the belly button, pulling your belly button in (squeezing in your abdominal muscles).

'Joining Joanna on her Walkactive Walk Firm course confirmed something I had suspected for some time: you do not need to spend hours in the gym or put your body under pressure to get results, fast. I have lost a total of 3 inches (7.5cm) off my midriff in four weeks. Walkactive works in a subtle yet hugely effective way, without putting strain on your body or your joints. I've toned virtually all my body. It is easy to maintain because Joanna rewires your brain to incorporate her method into your everyday life. For a woman in her fifties I haven't found another exercise routine that is so effective.'

TRACEY, 51, WALKACTIVE CLUB MEMBER

View Yourself From the Inside Out

Imagine you're standing in front of a full-length mirror with your clothes off. You want to see changes – whether that means inches off your waistline or beer belly, streamlined thighs, lifting and tightening of a saggy bum or simply dropping a size or two. But to achieve this, you have to stop obsessing about what you see in that mirror. Instead, I want you to shift your focus inward – to something you can't see. I know, it sounds crazy, but this is important! It's time to concentrate on what's happening in your body on a microscopic, cellular level. If you send the right messages to your cells, you will also see changes in the mirror, I guarantee it. In this chapter, I'm going to teach you how to communicate with your cells (through Walkactive, along with good nutrition), so that they use nutrients efficiently and burn off energy (calories). If you do this, you will have more energy and lose more inches!

Getting your head in the right place

If in the past you've tried – and failed – to 'lose weight', then you may already be undermining your plans without knowing it. There might be a little voice in your head saying, 'This won't work' or, 'This will work for a bit, then I'll quit – I always do.' Or perhaps you've decided to throw yourself into this heart and soul. Maybe you've had failures in the past, but this time you're absolutely determined. You're going to be *really* strict . . . See if you recognise yourself in the scenario below.

'My new diet'

Monday: a cup of black coffee and a piece of fruit for breakfast. A slim soup for lunch. A calorie-counted ready meal for supper. You take in a high-intensity fat-blaster aerobics class for good measure.

Tuesday: the same eating plan, but now you are starting to feel really hungry and deprived, as well as slightly snappy. You've been busy at your desk all day, but you haven't got up and moved around, so you drag yourself to the gym before treating yourself to your evening Ryvita and slim soup. You are exhausted, and a bit down.

Wednesday: you wake up decidedly craggy and short-tempered – you just about make it to the lunchtime Ryvita, but by 2pm you can't concentrate and you're craving sugar, so you grab a chocolate bar. The 'hit' makes you crave more sweet things. 'You know what? Stuff it!' you say. 'I've already blown it – might as well have another chocolate bar.' Then you have fish and chips and a glass of wine in front of the telly too. You go to bed feeling horrible. You've let yourself down so tomorrow you're going to be *extra*-good.

Thursday: no breakfast. Lunch is one measly Ryvita with a low-fat yoghurt (plus more caffeine – you're exhausted). You drag yourself to a spin class, but feel weak. You miserably have a slim soup for supper. You go to bed feeling down and starving.

Friday: another 'virtuous' day. But then it's 5pm – the weekend. You go out with friends and before you know it, you've downed two Margueritas and a plate of cheesy nachos. But you've been 'good' for almost two days, so you can 'afford' to treat yourself. The night turns into a 'blowout'. You feel bad. The number on the scales has barely changed. Why can't you stick to anything? You'll do better next week. Next week you'll be *really* good . . .

The 'all-or-nothing' approach probably seems to make sense – if you average out your calories over the week, they probably wouldn't be that excessive. But what makes sense to your brain makes absolutely no sense at all to your cells. They cannot use the nutrients and calories you give them if there are such massive fluctuations day to day. They get overloaded on the blowout days then go into 'starvation mode' – desperately trying to hold on to the energy (mostly as fat) when you don't eat.

We are going to erase this destructive (and demoralising) boom-bust behaviour once and for all. We'll focus on perfecting your Walkactive technique, being consistent with the plan and with my simple eating strategies. There will be no deprivation or calorie-counting. And you're not going to obsess about food or the bathroom scales. You're just going to eat sensibly – and walk!

Where are you now?

Before you start the plan it's important to establish your current average daily baseline (see page 75) and to take your measurements (see page 137). This will give you your starting point to measure your progress against. It's important to do this because as you see your steps increase and the inches dropping off, you will feel more motivated and confident that this is really working.

How to increase your daily steps

You are going to build up to 7500 steps a day. If your current baseline is way off this mark, build up gradually. Don't push yourself too hard too soon. I want you to see how achievable this is.

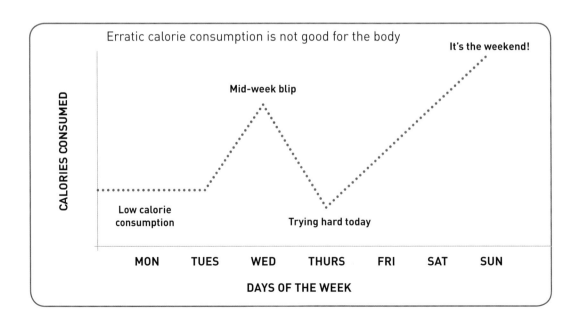

Erratic calorie consumption is not good for the body

CALORIES CONSUMED

It's the weekend!

Mid-week blip

Low calorie consumption

Trying hard today

MON   TUES   WED   THURS   FRI   SAT   SUN

DAYS OF THE WEEK

There are two ways of doing this. Choose the one that best fits your current activity pattern:

Option one

Your days are erratic – some days you walk a lot, others hardly at all. You currently average 5000 steps a day, but that might be made up of: day one – 1000 steps; day two – 11,000; day three – 3000.

What to do

Build up your step count gradually, by adding 500 steps per day. In week one add 500 steps per day for the next seven days, so you hit a baseline of 5500 every day. In week two raise your daily target a further 500, so you are hitting 6000 steps per day. Then repeat, adding 500 steps per week, until you are at 7500.

Option two

Your days are pretty much the same, but your step count is just way too low. So you are averaging, say, 5000 steps per day, and your step count is very similar each day. For instance: day one is 4500, day two 5500, day three 5000 and so on.

What to do

Build up faster, by adding 1000 steps per day. So in week one aim to add 1000 steps to your existing daily baseline (so if your daily baseline is 4000, try to walk 5000 steps daily for one week), in week two add another 1000 and continue to do this until you are averaging at least 7500 steps as your baseline.

This is not about pressing the STOP button of your life; it's about building Walkactive into your day – every day. And it's doable: thousands of people just like you have done this and seen amazing inch-loss results. You just have to plan – and persist.

Getting started with Pace Walks

If you are new to exercise, the Pace Walks (see page 64) can seem a little daunting. However, how long your Pace Walks last will depend on your starting point:

- **New to exercise**: make your Pace Walks at least five minutes long – this means your total Pace Walk, including warm-up and cool-down, takes around ten to twelve minutes to complete.
- **Established walker or exerciser**: make your Pace Walks at least fifteen minutes long (adding warm-up and cool-down to this time). But remember, this is just a guide. If you can't spare that much time, then shorter Pace Walks will do – just pay particular attention to your technique. You'll still see results with shorter walks, but if you aim for longer ones, you'll see results quicker.

Finding ways to walk when you're time short

There are two key factors in building Walkactive into your busy life and they are forward planning and options.

So first, I want you to have a think about your daily life: where do you go most frequently and regularly? Work? The school gates? The shops? Next, think about the routes you take to and from these places. If you plan a few different options – say, a five-, ten- and fifteen-minute route from your home to each of these – you can choose one, depending on how much time you have to spare. This will get more steps into your day – I guarantee it.

Use the chart above to plan out your route options (or use it as a template for your notebook). Include the following and/or any others you can think of:

- from home to the office
- from home to the school gates
- from home to your commute point (e.g. bus stop, Tube/train station)
- from home to the shops/supermarket
- from home to the pub(!)
- from home to a friend's house
- walking the dog

My routes

From:	To:
My 5-minute route	
My 10-minute route	
My 15-minute route	

One-off routes

You can also think about how you'll include walking when you go somewhere different. For instance, you know that tomorrow you'll be visiting an older relative, going to see a friend who's in hospital or travelling to a new part of town for a meeting. Here's where your planning skills come in. You need to work out how you'll fit a five-, ten- or fifteen-minute walk into tomorrow's route. This is a great way to up your daily step count without feeling inconvenienced or stressed.

The more you plan ahead and give yourself route options, the more your confidence and creativity will grow. You'll start incorporating Walkactive into more and more aspects of your life. This is by far the best way to increase your steps to 7500 every single day.

TROUBLESHOOTING

If you are overweight and new to Walkactive some of the following may sound familiar:

'My ankles hurt!' When you carry excess weight the tendency can be to have a passive foot and walk with a shuffle. You may feel some discomfort because your ankle is getting used to opening up. This is quite normal – it's all part of the process of connecting with your body, and using your full range of joint movement. So persevere. Focus on keeping your foot soft and pliable and your hips lifted.

 TIP *Mobilise your ankles before starting your Pace Walks*

Point your toes, then shift to press your heel down. Do this a few times. Circle your ankles two to three times on each leg before you start. This is a useful warm-up in cold weather, or if you drive to the place where you do your Walkactive. When you are driving your foot is flexed, and this can also contribute to shin discomfort when you start out. Similarly, if you spend all day at a desk, your ankles and feet will be used to being in a fixed ninety-degree angle. You want to mobilise those ankles as much as you can before you get going.

'My whole body aches!' The sensation of really using your body may be new to you.

To change your shape you have to put your body into what's called 'overload'. Overload stimulates your cells to adapt (see page 115), in order that you get fitter. So expect a bit of discomfort at first. However, if this discomfort is sharp or really painful, slow down! You have to build up gradually – and you will still see amazing results.

'My shins hurt!' Your weight usually falls into your pelvis, putting pressure on your knees. With Walkactive you are shifting your centre of gravity, and this can put pressure on your shins. The way to counter this pressure is to practise your Abdominal Js, so that your core gets stronger. Also, focus on your hip lift – lifting up from the knees and out of your hips.

Your miracle inch-loss tool: the Abdominal J

I've already waxed lyrical about my Abdominal Js (see page 37 for a full description), but if there's one exercise that really needs to become a part of your life it's this little beauty. Try to incorporate it into your walking, your Pace Walks and *your life* (doing the washing-up, standing in the supermarket queue, waiting for a bus . . . you get the picture). Just do your Abdominal Js whenever and wherever you can. They really will make a dramatic difference to your waistline.

Abdominal J variations

If you're getting bored with standard Abdominal Js, or you want a bit of a challenge, here are a few things to try:

- **Basic 10s** Do your Abdominal Js (standing), remembering it is a hold-in and drawing-up – you feel it starting deep down at the pubic bone and lengthening all the way up to your sternum. Hold for ten counts and release for ten. Repeat ten times.

- **Perfect Two Count** Do your Abdominal Js, holding for two slow counts and focusing on dropping the shoulders and drawing your ribcage down (this is an amazing waist-whittling movement, so don't be tempted to skip it). Visualise your Abdominal Js as being as perfect as possible on the last count. Release for five counts. Repeat five times.

- **Lengthening Pulses** These are fast-contraction Abdominal Js using a perfect technique. Make sure that your shoulders don't rise (remember that perfect physical oxymoron: abdominals in and up, ribcage and shoulders down). You are scooping in and under and up to your sternum, keeping your bottom relaxed. Lengthen with each contraction, then release. Repeat ten times.

- **Walking Abdominal Js** Do your basic Abdominal Js – drawing in and up and holding for ten – but this time do it as you walk. Take ten strides while holding your Abdominal J, then relax. Repeat eight to ten times (any more than this and your attention wanes and then you start to compromise your technique). Walking does make this more complicated and you might find that your pace eases off a bit, but that's fine – the main thing to focus on here is your Abdominal J technique.

- **Perfect Two Walking** Repeat the Perfect Two Count Abdominal Js, as with standing, but this time hold for two Walkactive strides, then release. Repeat as you walk 100m, then stop.

 Sifting flour

Imagine you have a big bowl of flour in front of you. Put your hands in the bowl and then scoop them out again. As you lift your hands, the flour sifts through your fingers. Try to get as much air into the flour as you can. It's that upward, scooping movement you're aiming for (while keeping ribcage and shoulders from rising up). In my experience many clients find it is really helpful to follow the J shape with their hands – especially in the early stages of mastering the technique. You may find the photographs on page 37 helpful.

GOOD NUTRITION: EATING FOR INCH LOSS

If you want to see really significant inch loss you also have to look at what you are eating. But don't worry. This isn't another faddy diet plan. I'm simply going to give you five easy-to-follow key strategies for good, sensible nutrition. Yes, calories are important, but calorie-counting can be extremely tedious. So I'm going to help you to cut down on excessive calories without obsessing or

'I attended Joanna's Introductory Walkactive One-day Workshop and, to be honest, I struggled with the pace sessions, as I really was not very fit. But I practised my technique daily, and when I went back to see Joanna two weeks later, I was amazed to find that I'd trimmed nearly 2 inches [5cm] off my waistline – without radically changing my diet! I was thrilled. I was not expecting results so quickly!'

VALERIE, 67, ATTENDED WALKACTIVE ONE-DAY WORKSHOP

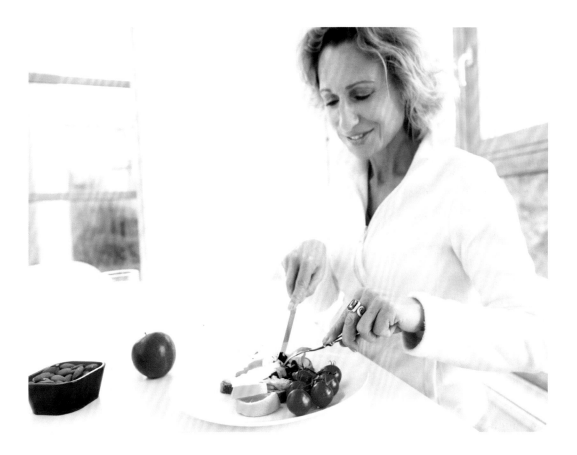

having to count anything. Follow these five sensible strategies and you *will* see results.

Strategy 1: the Carb Curfew

Carbs aren't 'bad' as such – in fact, the right kind of carbs, i.e. nutrient-rich wholemeal and wholegrains, rather than white-flour-based sugary foods – are an important part of any balanced diet; but they do sometimes contain hidden calories, often in the form of sugar (particularly in processed foods).

The Carb Curfew is not rocket science, but it works brilliantly. It's my number-one favourite nutrition tool. I first developed it when I was studying for my Masters degree, writing my thesis on body-composition change. My research showed me that when people became good at cutting out the fat in their diet, they often started to eat more carbohydrates. I also noticed that people who were (rightly) trying to eat more fibre also ate a lot of carbs without knowing it; they were therefore consuming too many calories.

The Carb Curfew is a simple way to control your calories while eating a nutritionally balanced diet. It means eating no starchy carbohydrates (bread, pasta, rice, potatoes or cereal) after 5pm. Don't panic though – you can incorporate a whole variety of nutritious foods into your evening meal, including lean meat and fish, fruit, vegetables, pulses and dairy products. It just takes a bit of planning.

The Carb Curfew Works Because...

· **It helps you control your blood-sugar levels**, stabilising your energy (you lose the 'sugar crashes').

· **It helps you cut calories** without having to count them.

· **It boosts your vitamin and mineral intake**: you are now eating fruit and vegetables instead of rice, pasta and potatoes.

· **It can reduce bloating**. Your body breaks carbohydrates down into glucose, storing it as glycogen in the muscles or as fat in the fat cells. Your body prefers to store these starchy carbohydrates as glycogen, but for every unit of glycogen it stores, it also has to store three units of water. Result? A bloated belly!

· **It stops 'food hangovers'**. If you stuff your face at night, you will wake up with a food hangover: you won't feel like eating breakfast, but by the evening you'll be starving again – and this is the point in the day when your willpower is at its lowest.

Strategy 2: avoid portion distortion

Don't fall into the trap of thinking: 'I'm so much more active, I can afford to eat more now!' Serving sizes have grown bigger and bigger and we are losing all sense of what a 'normal' or 'reduced' portion size really is. And excess food means excess calories, which, unless you burn them off, mean weight gain. Simple as that. So if you want to change your shape dramatically without feeling deprived, focus on your portion sizes. It's a brilliant way to keep excess calorie intake in check without calorie-counting or obsession. You can still enjoy a wide range of 'normal' foods. You simply control how much of them you eat.

Portion distortion checklist

Weighing food portions is a bore, so use my checklist instead:

Think . . .	for . . .
Two dice	nuts and cheese
A deck of cards	meat and fish
One teaspoon	oils and fats
A tennis ball	vegetables
A golf ball	uncooked rice or couscous
A computer mouse	a cooked portion of starchy carbs

Strategy 3: look at your 'food ratios'

I want you to try to improve the protein/carbohydrate balance in your meals – to do this, you will have to concentrate on eating more protein. Protein helps you to feel fuller for longer. It also stabilises your energy levels. I find that eating more protein at lunch keeps me switched on all afternoon, so I don't get that post-lunch energy slump. Also, eating fewer carbs at lunch will keep your body temperature lower – again, this guards against the afternoon 'crash'.

All you have to do is eat an equal amount of protein and carbohydrate at lunchtime. To keep it simple, just work it out visually. For instance, a ham sandwich made of two slices of bread (carbs) and one slice ham (protein) has a carb/protein ratio of 2:1. Swap this for an open salad sandwich made of one slice bread (carbs), some salad and top with sliced ham (protein). This gives you a ratio of 1:1, and you still have a tasty, satisfying lunch.

I know it can be hard to make a big change if you are used to eating lots of carbs, but this is a habit and, as such, it can be broken. It's a question of keeping going until eating fewer carbs becomes second nature – in fact, you'll find you no longer crave carbs as you used to.

Why look at food ratios?

- Protein contains leucine – an essential amino acid that is important for building lean muscles. Your body cannot produce leucine naturally, so you have to get it from food. Studies show that leucine doesn't just preserve lean muscle tissue, it may also promote fat loss.
- Whereas carbs, particularly when refined, will give you an energy spike followed by an energy 'crash' where you – yes – crave more carbs/sugar, protein guards against a steep rise in blood sugar after a meal or snack.
- Protein stimulates the release of dopamine, a brain transmitter that actually makes you feel more alert, boosting concentration and curbing lethargy. Again, this lowers the sugary-snack temptation.

Strategy 4: eat less fat

A gram of fat contains more than double the calories of a gram of protein or carbohydrate. Cutting down on saturated ('bad') fats not only helps to keep your calories in check, it also protects your cardiovascular health. Try to cut down dramatically on saturated fats, such as full-fat dairy products, fatty meats or sugary foods, such as cakes, chocolate and cookies. However don't be fooled by 'low-fat' and 'fat-free' labels on products – this can often mean that the food has added sugar, so look at the full ingredients list.

 TIP   *Do eat small amounts of good fats*

I'm actually a fan of fats – as long as they are good fats! Good fats are heart-healthy, and it's important to include them in your diet. They are found in foods such as avocados, nuts and some oils (such as olive, vegetable, sunflower or rapeseed oil). However, when you include good fats in your diet, do so in moderation – bear in mind portion distortion. They are still fats and, as such, they are calorie-dense.

Why eat less fat?

- Research shows that lowering dietary fat helps you lose weight because you simply take in fewer calories.
- High-fat foods are often not as filling: they stimulate cravings and make it harder to not overeat.

Strategy 5: breakfast – front-load your day

Starving yourself early in the day, with the notion that you are saving calories, is a false economy. It only leads to stress, hunger, cravings and overeating at night. Eating a good breakfast that includes some protein as well as carbs to stabilise your energy is therefore really important. But if you can't face food first thing, don't worry – any time up to 11am will do the trick. Just make sure it is healthy and not a double espresso and gooey pastry!

What About Alcohol?

You don't have to give up alcohol entirely, but you should limit your intake. Try to aim for no more than one to two units (a unit being a small glass of wine or one shot of spirits) a night – but, as always, saving your nightly 'quota' for a weekend binge is not a great idea. This will give you a surge in calories and stop your aim of consistency. Complete abstinence is great, if you can do that – or simply cut it out during the week and have a unit or two at the weekend or on a special occasion.

Why limit alcoholic drinks?

- Alcohol is high in calories. These calories cannot be used directly by your muscles – instead they go straight into your bloodstream, where they are converted into fuel sources such as fat and glycogen, and stored – that is, as fat. Research suggests that for this reason, alcohol may be worse for your waistline than a slice of cake with the same calorie content (which could, in theory, be used up directly by your muscles).

- Alcohol weakens your willpower – it's harder to make good choices when you're a bit squiffy.

- Alcohol leaves you less satisfied by food: a study published in the *American Journal of Clinical Nutrition* found that drinking a single glass of wine or beer before lunch leaves you less satisfied after the meal and increases the chances that you'll eat more over the next twenty-four hours.

Why eat breakfast?

- It helps to stabilise your energy levels.
- It regulates appetite. If you wait until later, when you are starving, you will find it harder to make sensible food choices, and when you do eat again you'll find it harder to recognise when you are full.
- It provides your body with energy when it needs it, rather than at the end of the day, when you are generally less active. There's a lot to be said for the old adage: breakfast like a king, lunch like a prince and dine like a pauper.

 TIP   *Be consistent*

Consistency is the key to creating the optimum environment for your cells. Ideally, to maximise your body's use of energy from food, you should aim to eat roughly the same amount of food every day. This means you should not binge one day, then starve the next to make up for it. And the good thing about my eating strategies is that they make this easy for you. It's all about losing the panic, sticking to the strategies and aiming for common sense and consistency above all.

TIP ···

Drink more water

Drinking more water every day can make you feel amazing. Again and again I see people not hydrating effectively – and even if they do drink the recommended quota of 1.2 litres a day (about eight glasses), they do so by glugging it down in one go rather than drinking little and often. Imagine your body is a house plant; if you haven't watered it for a week, then you come home and slosh a load of water in, you'll find that it can't absorb that much liquid. Water seeps out the bottom of the plant pot and the plant will still look a little sorry for itself. If, on the other hand, you water that plant little and often it will use the water properly, and look healthy and perky. Our bodies work in the same way.

A handy tip to remind you to drink water is to have two small pots next to each other on your desk or in your kitchen, one containing eight pebbles, the other empty. Each pebble represents a glass of water. Every time you finish a glass of water, move one pebble across from the full pot to the empty one, until all the pebbles have been moved. Aim to move three pebbles by lunchtime, another three by the end of the afternoon, and the last two by the time you go to bed. You'll feel a radical difference to your energy levels, I promise.

How to eat healthily all day

This is a great way to approach your daily nutrition. I'm not suggesting you eat the same thing every day – I'm just giving you an idea of what you're aiming for.

Breakfast

You are aiming to:

- become more alert and fuel yourself with energy for the morning
- eat some protein and a small amount of carbohydrate.

Try

- poached egg on toast and a glass of fresh fruit juice, or
- wholegrain toast with nut butter (try white almond butter for luxurious tasting 'good' fats) and sliced apple on top.

Lunch

You are aiming to:

- head off a post-lunch slump by eating food ratio 1:1 (see page 147)
- boost brainpower and energy for the afternoon, and keep sugar cravings away.

Try

- an open chicken salad sandwich, or
- gazpacho garnished with chopped egg and some cottage cheese with chopped cucumber, peppers and avocado, served with a small slice of rye bread.

If you're buying lunch on the go, try to find options such as salads and soups with less bread, more protein (or, even, discard the top slice of bread on a bought sandwich).

Afternoon snack

You are aiming to:

- keep your spirits lifted and stop that 'get-home-ravenous' feeling
- rehydrate and keep your brain in gear.

Try

- if you're a milk lover, a large glass of skimmed milk with ice; this will give you a protein blast and an essential calcium kick (you could add a square of 70 per cent dark chocolate for a mood-boosting antioxidant punch), or
- if you don't like milk, try an oatcake with hummus or nut butter plus a small glass of fruit juice diluted to make about 500–750ml (drink this gradually through the afternoon).

Dinner

You are aiming to:

- release tension without going to bed stuffed.

Try

- a quick grab-on-the-way-home option in the form of a bag of salad leaves and a roasted chicken; depending on

time, fortify the salad bag with other raw vegetables (carrot ribbons, baby tomatoes, cucumber, mixed fresh herbs, steamed broccoli, sautéed mushrooms in a little Thai sweet chilli sauce) and top with the warm roasted chicken strips, or

- make an easy swap to enjoy a 'Carb Curfew spaghetti Bolognese' – just substitute the pasta with a delicious mound of courgette ribbons, steamed for one minute and served with Bolognese sauce; quick, easy and incredibly nutritious.

 Soup to the rescue

If you often get home starving hungry, having a tomato-based vegetable soup to hand is a great help. This will stop you snacking on ill-advised foods or overeating at dinner. It also gives you vegetables and hydration. But remember the Carb Curfew so no bread, pasta, rice, potatoes or cereal with or in the soup.

What about eating in the real world?

Of course it can be hard to put all these principles into practice all the time, when even the best-laid plans can be scuppered by a social life. Here's my guide to making it work:

Suggested strategy for balancing your meals

	Day 1	Day 2	Day 3	Day 4	Day 5	Day 6	Day 7
Breakfast	As recommended	As recommended	As recommended	As recommended	As recommended	As recommended	As recommended
Lunch	Food ratio	Food ratio	Carb-free zone	Carb-free zone	Carb-free zone	Food ratio	Carb-free zone
Snack	As recommended	As recommended	As recommended	As recommended	As recommended	As recommended	As recommended
Dinner	Carb Curfew	Carb Curfew	Dinner at friends	As recommended	Carb Curfew	Meal at restaurant	Carb Curfew
Calorie range	Calorie range stable with 300–400 calorie maximum variation						

- The Carb Curfew – easiest to use when you're cooking for yourself and can plan and eat the way you want. But you may also be able to make Carb-Curfew restaurant choices too.
- Try a carb-free zone on days when you're eating out (going to dinner at a friend's house, for instance) and you know you may not be able to avoid eating carbs. You simply switch your day around – so that lunch or breakfast are carb-free instead of dinner.
- Apply portion-distortion principles to your sociable dining – so when you go out, do enjoy your meal, be a good guest, but don't eat everything on your plate. Remember my portion-distortion checklist and use it.
- Don't forget forward planning. If you have a sociable weekend ahead, try to limit your carb intake for the two days beforehand. Don't limit your food so much that you feel starved or deprived (if you do that, you'll only end up wolfing down too much food at the weekend). However, on Thursday or Friday try to: eat no carbs at lunch or dinner; be rigorous about portion control and stick to the strategic mid-afternoon snack (or the homecoming cup of soup). Then, on the weekend itself: include protein at breakfast; drink at least 1 litre of water (in four glasses) by noon; and operate a Carb Curfew or carb-free zone, depending on what's practical.

Carb Curfew or Carb-free Zone?

The regular evening Carb Curfew is the more effective strategy of the two, so try to aim for this wherever possible. And think of the movable carb-free zone as your back-up plan; it's much better to do this than to simply ignore the issue altogether and eat carbs at all meals.

CASE STUDY: KAREN – SHAPE CHANGE

Karen, aged forty-five, was extremely overweight and had long believed that exercise was something she could only try if she lost a lot of weight first. It took some courage for her to come to my Walkactive Walk off Weight Camp, but she realised that since she has to walk every day anyway, it might just work.

'I was anxious before I went to camp,' she says. 'I was worried that I wouldn't be able to do what everyone else could do, worried I wouldn't be pushed and, most importantly, worried I wouldn't try hard enough . . . I did find the course tough, but although I was last on every event, I never once felt I was last. Instead, I felt I'd succeeded by completing the challenge.'

Buoyed up by the support and encouragement of the group, Karen began to see that change was possible. 'I was getting stronger – and, bit by bit, my negative beliefs were being chipped away.' Karen says that she came home from the camp 'a different person'.

'I walk taller and I can feel the changes in my body,' she says. 'By lengthening my stride and using my arms, I've reduced my waist, my neck feels longer and my joints are more flexible. I can see my shape returning. I have more energy and therefore I'm even more active. I actively look for opportunities to walk now.'

Since coming home, Karen has introduced my eating strategies – she aims to keep her calories consistent through the week, and has virtually stopped eating carbs in the evening. She also works hard to drink lots of water. She has lost 10lb (4.5kg) and 11 inches (28cm).

'The biggest difference is inside my head,' she says. 'Now, I am much better at overcoming the weak or absent-minded moments where I want to eat something that I shouldn't. I tell myself it's the equivalent of a 3km walk. And if I'm thinking I can't do something, I remind myself that I did an 11km walk up a mountain – I can then persuade myself to give it a go or try harder.'

Karen plans to sign up for Walk Time Trials. There is no going back now – she's found her path to a healthy shape. 'I know,' she says, 'that I'm going to succeed!'

YOUR TWELVE-WEEK WALKACTIVE FOR INCH-LOSS PLAN

To help you put all this advice into practice here is a suggested inch-loss plan. If at any time you find this too easy or too difficult simply adjust the length of your Pace Walks accordingly but do ensure you follow the basic inch-loss plan – that is to:

1. Raise your daily baseline to 7500 steps every day
2. Complete four Pace Walks each week
3. Complete my Carb Curfew on five out of seven days

As with the Fitness Plan in the previous chapter, I've divided my Inch-loss Plan into three phases: it will be easier to follow if you break it down.

Phase One: stop the rot

Your aim by day twenty-eight is to:

Weeks one to four	• Complete the fitness test (see page 116) and record results – do this right at the start of day 1 so you get a true measure to compare against
	• Build your daily baseline to 7500 steps, and consolidate this – aim to have your daily baseline at 7500 by day 14, then from day 14 on you are consolidating
	• Complete your four Pace Walks a week (perform your Abdominal Js on these sessions); aim to build up from five to twelve minutes
	• Introduce one 'One route – three ways' session (see page 120)
	• Aim to complete two 'Slopes-and-stride' sessions (see page 121)
	• Get a Walk Time Trial (see page 126) completed – at the end of Week 4.
	• Ideally I'd like you to start to implement my Carb Curfew – experiment with it three times a week or build up to five times a week if you feel ready for it. However, if trying to achieve your walking targets and your Carb Curfew target is a bridge too far right now leave it to Phase Two but try to introduce as many of the other eating strategies as you can

Phase Two: building confidence

Your aim by day fifty-six is to:

Weeks five to eight	• Confidently achieve a minimum baseline of 7500 steps every day
	• Complete four Pace Walks per week (perform your Abdominal Js in these sessions and feel stronger doing them); these should now be building up to at least fifteen minutes and ideally forty minutes in duration
	• Add variety to your Pace Walks by making three of these 'Slopes-and-stride' sessions
	• Do two '4 x 10' sessions (see page 125)
	• Do one 'One route – three ways' session
	• Add a Walk Time Trial to help track your progress at the end of Week 7
	• If you deferred trying your Carb Curfew in Phase One aim in this block to enforce a Carb Curfew three to four times a week. If you already have Carb Curfew cracked – aim to consistently do this five out of seven nights a week, and if you really want to experiment completing it for seven consecutive evenings

Phase Three: putting it all together

Your aim by day eighty-four is to:

Weeks nine to twelve	• Consistently achieve 7500 daily steps, and complete four Pace Walks a week with Abdominal Js
	• Up the intensity by adding two '4 x 12' sessions to your Pace Walks
	• Complete one 'Slopes-and-stride' session each week
	• Make your Carb Curfew five to seven nights a week a regular feature of your daily eating plan – and follow the other four points of the eating strategy too
	• Complete a Walk Time Trial in your final week, and record your time

A word of advice: shhhhhhhh

With the best will in the world, some people will try to sabotage your efforts if you tell them you're on a new 'healthy-eating' plan. This is why, in my experience, it's often best not to talk about the changes you're making. Simply use the strategies outlined in this chapter and enjoy your meals with friends, without discussing what you're doing.

MONITORING YOUR PROGRESS

I recommend measuring yourself once a week. This will give you a sense of progress, and that's really important for your motivation and success. Alternatively, you could choose one pair of jeans that you put on once a week – you'll notice them getting looser!

My clients have lost up to 10 inches (25cm) in four weeks, but it's important to be aware that people see different rates of 'shrinkage'. Try not to get obsessed: just keep with the plan and be confident that you too are going to lose inches and see a transformation. It *will* happen if you consistently stick to the plan.

MAINTAINING YOUR NEW SHAPE

Once you reach your target, you need to make sure that you maintain this amazing new you. And this is what people mean when they say that Walkactive is a lifestyle choice. I don't want you to simply go back to walking a few thousand steps a day and eating all the carbs you like. If you do this, you know what's going to happen! Instead, I want you to think of Walkactive as a lifetime habit: to maintain your daily 7500 steps and aim for three Pace Walks a week. I also want you to keep up your Carb Curfew about 80 per cent of the time. My eating strategies are all strategies for life: portion distortion, protein ratios, fat control all make for healthy, balanced eating (that liberates you from fussy, faddy diets). By now they should be your habits – and, as such, they should be easy to maintain.

None of this should be painful. This plan is sustainable, healthy, simple, enjoyable – and best of all, it really works. With my approach to nutrition you can enjoy the odd treat and eat a full and interesting range of foods. This isn't a diet or a 'regime' – it's a way of life. In short, with Walkactive for Inch Loss you can live your life to the full, while maintaining – and loving! – an incredible new shape. For ever.

CONCLUSION

I'm completely passionate about what I do.

When I see the incredible changes that Walkactive brings, I know without any doubt that it works – in fact sometimes it works miracles. Whether it's an elderly man regaining his mobility and independence, a fitness fanatic increasing her cardiovascular fitness, a young woman gaining body confidence, a busy executive shedding inches, a celebrity who looks a million dollars on the red carpet – or any number of my clients who have lost inches, now enjoy pain-free exercise, grown fitter, healthier, more confident, lean and strong – these amazing results are what motivate me to spring out of bed in the morning. These transformations confirm what I already know scientifically: that Walkactive is a highly effective technique – for any body.

Walkactive has grown and evolved from my study of movement, fitness and the human body for over twenty years. I have worked with thousands of people – people just like you – who now benefit massively from something they do every day. What's more, I have seen how Walkactive is transferred across all aspects of their lives, bringing not just physical, but emotional and lifestyle transformations too. My clients gain confidence, they find love or new careers; they make new friends, climb mountains (sometimes literally), speak out, move on – change their lives.

Walkactive is just so simple. It makes perfect physiological sense. It's sustainable and practical. It brings dramatic results. It's free. It's liberating. It's fun. And now it's your turn! Whatever your personal circumstances, goals or challenges Walkactive will work for you – if you let it.

So, it's time to put one foot in front of the other. You can do this. Go for it!

Joanna x

INDEX

Note: page numbers in **bold** refer to diagrams and photographs, page numbers in *italics* refer to information contained in tables.